Antipsychotics and their Side Effects

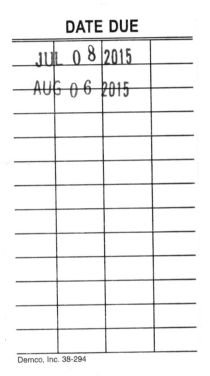

Antipsychotics and their Side Effects

David M. Gardner

Professor of Psychiatry
Department of Psychiatry and College of Pharmacy
Dalhousie University, Halifax, Canada

Michael D. Teehan

Associate Professor
Department of Psychiatry
Dalhousie University, Halifax, Canada

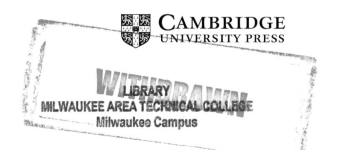

CAMBRIDGE
UNIVERSITY PRESS

CAMBRIDGE UNIVERSITY PRESS

Cambridge, New York, Melbourne, Madrid, Cape Town, Singapore, São Paulo, Delhi, Dubai, Tokyo, Mexico City

Cambridge University Press
The Edinburgh Building, Cambridge CB2 8RU, UK

Published in the United States of America by Cambridge University Press, New York

www.cambridge.org
Information on this title: www.cambridge.org/9780521132084

First published 2011

Printed in the United Kingdom at the University Press, Cambridge

A catalog record for this publication is available from the British Library

ISBN 978-0-521-13208-4 Paperback

Additional resources for this publication at www.cambridge.org/9780521132084

We dedicate this book first and foremost to people, patients, and families affected by mental illness. It is also dedicated to those who direct their energy, knowledge, and skills to advocate and care for them.

Contents

Foreword

Antipsychotics and their Side Effects is authored by Professor David M. Gardner, Department of Psychiatry and College of Pharmacy, and Associate Professor Michael D. Teehan, Department of Psychiatry, Dalhousie University, Halifax, Canada. The authors are highly experienced clinicians with strong academic interests that include expert knowledge of antipsychotic drugs. Their book is divided into three sections: (i) 20 chapters with references and tables on adverse effects of antipsychotic drugs (including hematological, anticholinergic, metabolic, neurological, ophthalmological, cardiovascular, dermatological, sexual, and urinary effects, and changes in vital signs), emphasizing the adverse effects in relation to specific drugs, with tabulated recommendations about monitoring; (ii) tabulated specific recommendations and guidelines for monitoring individual drugs (aripiprazole, chlorpromazine, clozapine, flupenthixol, fluphenazine, haloperidol, loxapine, methotrimeprazine, molindone, olanzapine, paliperidone, pericyazine, perphenazine, pimozide, pipotiazine palmitate, quetiapine, risperidone, thioridazine, thiothixene, trifluoperazine, ziprasidone, and zuclopenthixol); and (iii) guidelines for eliciting information from patients, including the use of novel assessment forms to monitor for adverse effects during treatment with antipsychotic drugs, with the implicit aims of limiting risk of adverse effects and facilitating timely clinical interventions. The material compiled is solidly grounded on findings from the research literature.

A major motivation for writing this book is the authors' stated impression that the second-generation antipsychotic drugs have brought limited clinical advances in efficacy for the treatment of psychotic, manic, and other disorders over the first-generation neuroleptics that have entered clinical psychiatry since the early 1950s, although with dissimilar patterns of adverse effects. The newer antipsychotics brought variable reductions in risk of some adverse neurological effects but their own set of complex metabolic and other risks. In turn, Drs. Gardner and Teehan call for dealing with this complexity by particularly active and thoughtful monitoring for a broad spectrum of adverse effects that are addressed systematically in this book. Their approach is particularly timely, as contemporary clinical psychiatry – no doubt encouraged by the substantial, if partial, success of pharmacological treatments for many disorders – appears to be tending increasingly to devalue traditional clinical skills, with the risk of more brief, superficial, and technical approaches to clinical therapeutics. Interactions with patients sometimes seem surprisingly impersonal and far from psychiatry's tradition of centering the patient–clinician interaction on the views and experiences of individual patients. This book should contribute to limiting such trends.

The modern era of clinical psychopharmacology can be dated from the introduction of lithium carbonate for mania and then for long-term prophylaxis in manic-depressive (bipolar) disorder in the late 1940s, and of chlorpromazine for the treatment of mania and acute psychosis, and later for chronic psychotic disorders including schizophrenia in the early 1950s. These largely serendipitous advances initiated major, even revolutionary, changes in psychiatric diagnostics as well as therapeutics [1]. However, the story of modern antipsychotic drugs only in part is about scientific innovation and rational application of principles arising from basic neuroscience, neuropharmacology, medicinal chemistry, and rational therapeutic experimentation [1–3]. In addition, it is characterized by powerful sociological trends. These include a degree of wishful overvaluing of the new treatments, and of disinclination to face squarely the limitations and considerable clinical problems associated with this class of palliative drugs. Even such terms as "side effect" and "atypical" with respect to antipsychotic drugs are problematic, and euphemistically suggest occasional minor costs to be balanced against consistent major clinical benefits.

In reality, the benefits of antipsychotic drug treatments often are modest, at least in chronic psychotic disorders including schizophrenia, delusional disorders,

schizoaffective conditions, and in the dementias. Even their more striking benefits in mania and acute psychotic syndromes typically require weeks or even months for full symptomatic remission, and they often fail to provide substantial benefit for cognitive and functional status at any time. In turn, this is a story of business and marketing in a multibillion dollar per year industry. Importantly, all of these developments have had an important impact on the shaping of modern psychiatric practice, with growing emphasis on standardization and purported "efficiency," largely driven by a desire to limit clinician time and costs. In a more salutary direction, the book further implies that the range and complexity of adverse clinical effects of antipsychotic and other psychotropic agents encourage renewed interest in general medicine among psychiatric clinicians.

It is to be hoped that choices of drugs, doses, timing, and duration of treatment would arise primarily from the clinically interpreted outcomes of randomized, controlled, and well-designed and managed clinical trials. However, for now, such evidence with respect to the antipsychotic drugs is very limited. With the probable and still-unexplained exception of clozapine (an older drug, first patented in 1960), most older and newer antipsychotic drugs are indistinguishable from one another with respect to efficacy in short-term controlled trials, or in long-term clinical effectiveness. All antipsychotics currently employed clinically or commercially have passed regulatory requirements of showing evidence of some degree of efficacy or statistical superiority to a placebo or no active treatment. Sometimes, the benefits are only a few percentage points above outcomes associated with a placebo: statistically "significant," but often of marginal clinical superiority, particularly in the continued or even new treatment of chronic psychotic disorders including schizophrenia. It remains extremely challenging to rank specific drugs by their likelihood or degree of clinical benefits. Although older and newer antipsychotics are remarkably similar in efficacy, the newer and far more expensive agents have been marketed aggressively and very successfully. Most of them do have substantially or even markedly reduced risks of certain adverse neurological effects, particularly acute dystonias, parkinsonism, and perhaps tardive dyskinesia, with continued risk of akathisia, but less or altered presentations of neuroleptic malignant syndrome as delirium and unstable vital signs, but far less muscle rigidity than with most first-generation neuroleptics [1].

In addition, the substantial but limited efficacy of most psychotropic drugs, coupled with powerful but often exaggerated iatrogenic expectations supporting their use, has encouraged increasingly complex and largely non-rational, or at least untested and unproved, applications of combinations and higher doses of drugs, including the antipsychotics. In turn, these trends can increase risks of sometimes unpredicted drug interactions and of adverse effects, even when individual drugs are prescribed at moderate doses [4,5].

An important theme of this book is that the important but partial benefits of the antipsychotic drugs as a class need to be balanced against their considerable risk of adverse metabolic, neurological, and other unwanted general medical effects [5,6]. It is particularly ironic that some of the most effective antipsychotic agents, such as clozapine and olanzapine, are complicated by a range of potentially severe or even life-threatening adverse medical effects. In the absence of clear, evidence-based differences in efficacy of most antipsychotics, such adverse-effect risks can usefully guide selection of drugs and doses for individual patients, with the aim of limiting risks. These risks range from the clinically incidental to severely uncomfortable, sometimes disabling, and occasionally lethal effects. The search continues for a scientific basis of rational psychiatric therapeutics based on research evidence of differences in efficacy among specific drugs, as a component of "evidence-based medicine." Progress to that aim would be greatly facilitated by head-to-head, direct, randomized comparisons of different agents or doses to test comparative efficacy directly. However, for now, individualized assessments of the impact of adverse effects, and the large variance in acquisition costs of individual drugs, arguably, are more significant factors in drug selection than differences in efficacy.

In short, the often minor or subtle differences in clinical benefits among specific antipsychotics make adequate understanding of the nature, recognition, and avoidance or amelioration of their adverse effects all the more important. Selection of drugs and doses that are well tolerated by individual patients is highly dependent on an informed clinician, alert to emerging signs and symptoms and, perhaps most important, of subjective distress that requires some effort and attention to elicit from each patient. These downsides of the clinical use of this important class of psychotropic drug are addressed comprehensively, thoughtfully, and critically by this book. In short, it is a valuable and timely teaching and reference work.

Ross J. Baldessarini, MD

Professor of Psychiatry and in Neuroscience,
Harvard Medical School
Director, Psychopharmacology Program,
McLean Hospital
Senior Consulting Psychiatrist, Massachusetts
General Hospital
Boston, MA, USA
April, 2010

REFERENCES

1. Baldessarini RJ, Tarazi FI. Pharmacotherapy of psychosis and mania. In Brunton LL, Lazo JS, Parker KL, eds., *Goodman and Gilman's The Pharmacological Basis of Therapeutics*, 11th edn. New York: McGraw-Hill; 2006.

2. Gardner DM, Baldessarini RJ, Waraich P. Modern antipsychotic agents: a critical overview. *Can Med Assoc J* 2005;**172**(13):1703–11.

3. Leucht S, Arbter D, Engel RR, Kissling W, Davis JM. How effective are second-generation antipsychotic drugs? A meta-analysis of placebo-controlled trials. *Mol Psychiatry* 2009;**14**(4):429–47.

4. Gardner DM, Murphy AL, O'Donnell H, Centorrino F, Baldessarini RJ. International consensus study of antipsychotic dosing. *Am J Psychiatry* 2010;**167**(6):686–693.

5. Centorrino F, Ventriglio A, Vincenti A, Talamo A, Baldessarini RJ. Changes in medication practices for hospitalized psychiatric patients: 2009 versus 2004. *Hum Psychopharmacol* 2010;**25**(2):179–86.

6. Bhuvaneswar C, Alpert J, Harsh V, Baldessarini RJ. Adverse endocrine and metabolic effects of psychotropic drugs. *CNS Drugs* 2009;**23**(12):1003–21.

Preface

The impetus to writing this book was, at first, local. In our academic center, psychiatrists and other clinicians involved in caring for patients with mental illnesses were in a quandary. The first wave of enthusiasm coming from the introduction of a new generation of antipsychotic medication was ebbing. The relief experienced in prescribing antipsychotics relatively free of the specter of disabling movement disorders was being tempered by new concerns. *Time* magazine cover stories and the marketing arms of pharmaceutical companies had fuelled expectations that were sagging in the face of clinical experience. Clinical trials of limited scope, some with overt biases in their design and analyses, were being more closely scrutinized and reconsidered. Critical appraisal of the whole field was raising disturbing questions about the measurable benefits from the introduction of expensive replacements for first-generation (conventional) antipsychotics. The increasingly irreconcilable claims of Pharma-sponsored work, research findings from publicly sponsored trials, and clinical experience created not only confusion but disappointment among clinicians in the trenches.

There were nagging questions in the air. Had we prematurely abandoned some very effective and trusted remedies, imperfect as they were? Did the new agents truly improve the quality of our patients' lives? Was the difference, if any, from the effects of the older agents worth the considerable increase in cost to the healthcare system and to our patients? Most worrying of all to clinicians was the question of whether we had substituted an equally damaging set of side effects for the familiar hazards of haloperidol and chlorpromazine.

There is a well described arc of activity with the introduction of new pharmaceuticals to the marketplace. Initial expectations drive a surge of switches from current treatment in resistant cases, and desperation promotes off-label use. This novelty phase begins to fade as failure of the new drug in poorly selected uses inevitably disappoints. The emergence of unexpected adverse events, not anticipated by the limited samples in clinical trials, emerges concurrently. Clinicians begin to focus selection of the new drug more finely and are more watchful for newly recognized adverse effects. At this point, growth in use of the medication is resumed but at a more measured pace. After several years, a niche is eventually found for the new agent.

We began to write these guidelines for monitoring antipsychotics at the end of the first wave of use. Clinicians have not found the second-generation (atypical) antipsychotics to be transformative for their patients. They do not improve the lives of all patients, and in some instances they worsen outcomes. The reality of a new set of adverse effects has become painfully obvious.

On the other hand, many patients have responded very well and have found the new medications to be more acceptable than their older treatment. The risk of acute, frightening extrapyramidal dysfunction in the early phase of treatment has been markedly but not entirely eliminated. Eventually, most patients were stabilized on their new regimens and were somewhat content with the change.

For many seasoned clinicians, however, simplicity had exited the scene. The comfort of defaulting to the same options among the original agents, which had spanned two generations of prescribers, had been replaced with the uncertainty of choice and with it a new set of concerns. The careful monitoring of treatment, with most attention focused on movement disturbances, no longer sufficed. A whole new area of concern had sent clinicians scrambling to retrieve their general medicine texts and to update themselves about metabolic disorders that had last concerned them as interns. It became clear to many that the physical health of their patients was suffering and their care was falling through the cracks. What should be monitored, how, when, and most importantly who should do

it have become questions challenging all who care for patients using antipsychotics.

As new concerns about the metabolic and other effects of the newer agents grew, older concerns faded and with them so did the skills of detection and treatment. New practitioners have rarely been exposed to the once common features of antipsychotic use. Senior residents report that they have seen very few cases of cogwheel rigidity and doubt if they could efficiently and effectively complete a standard physical assessment for the extremely well-characterized neurological adverse effects of antipsychotics. New practitioners have said that they were never taught these skills and experienced practitioners acknowledge that they are losing or no longer using them.

The end result for patients of the switch in prescribing trends, from first- to second-generation antipsychotics, is that they are being followed within a broken monitoring system that desperately needs remediation. Older, well-developed skills of assessment and monitoring need to be revitalized and at the same time new practices need to be implemented such that the safe and effective use of older and newer antipsychotics can be optimized.

Communications and planning merit special attention. Knowing how to detect and monitor antipsychotic side effects is not enough. Many patients see several physicians and other healthcare providers who are capable of monitoring their response to antipsychotics. Determining who is responsible for what, when it comes to monitoring patients taking antipsychotics, requires planning and ongoing communications among the patient's healthcare providers. Without this important clarification, systemic problems will not be resolved.

Our textbook will not address, let alone resolve, the many systemic challenges. However, it can serve as an accessible and informative resource of what to do, when to do it, and how to do it. It is designed to be a reference tool and to facilitate decision-making for optimal monitoring for people who are prescribed antipsychotic medications. We recognize the practical impediments to fully upholding these expectations (gaps in knowledge, lack of capable personnel, unwilling patients, time constraints, and fiscal limits). While acknowledging these challenges, we have tried to identify, describe, and guide comprehensive monitoring of clinically relevant adverse effects of antipsychotics. As is the practice in many areas of medicine, systematic monitoring provides the greatest safeguards. We propose a structured follow-up plan in each case, using standard measures, applied at defined intervals, to detect adverse effects and to monitor them regularly. The aim is to provide clinicians with a means of providing optimal, safety-oriented care to patients who are followed over lengthy periods. Who carries out this work and how it is done, we entrust to you.

Acknowledgements

This book represents the culmination of several years of effort and important contributions by numerous individuals. Approximately 6 years ago, recognizing the poor overall follow-up care that many of our patients were receiving, we embarked on a project as co-chairs to develop a comprehensive monitoring guide for Nova Scotia's Capital District Health Authority (CDHA). The aim of the guide was to improve the monitoring of patients, hospitalized and ambulatory, who were being treated with antipsychotic medications long term. Many of the ideas generated while developing the antipsychotic monitoring guide are reflected in this book and our gratitude goes to those who supported the development of the monitoring guide. Dr. S. Devarajan, Julie Garnham, Susan MacLellan, Dr. Heather Milliken, and Barbara O'Neill were members of the steering committee for the project, and Christopher Daley, Derek Roberts, Sheri Axworthy, Loa Barendregt, Fady Kamel, Christopher Dolan, Kathy Ann Turner, and Rochelle Myers, who were pharmacy and medical students at Dalhousie University and the University of Toronto, provided research assistance in the development of the CDHA monitoring guide. Without their dedicated and industrious help to the CDHA project, this book would never have materialized. During the final year of her psychiatry residency, Dr. Linda Hoyt developed the initial simplified antipsychotic monitoring form, which was tested with the cooperation of Dr. Edward Gordon and inpatient staff and patients. An updated version of this form can be found in this book. Financial support for the CDHA monitoring guide was provided by means of arms-length, unrestricted educational grants from multiple pharmaceutical companies including AstraZeneca, Janssen-Ortho, Eli Lilly, Novartis, and

Pfizer. Employees from these companies had no role in the content of the monitoring guide, nor have they provided any input towards the content of this book.

Melissa Hawkins, our book's final research assistant, provided the organizational, technical, and proofing skills we needed to complete this book. We would like to thank the Department of Health's Drug Evaluation Alliance of Nova Scotia (DEANS) program for their funding of Melissa's position. We also thank Drs. Andrea Murphy (Halifax, NS) and Karen Hoar (Mill Bay, BC) for their reviews and constructive feedback.

Purpose, development, and limitations of *Antipsychotics and their Side Effects*

Purpose

The possible side effects of antipsychotics are extensive, varied, frequently intolerable, too often serious, and sometimes fatal. Clinicians cannot be expected to use these drugs optimally in the care of their patients when inexperienced with the antipsychotic prescribed or unfamiliar with the adverse possibilities and how to monitor for them. This book aims to support clinicians in improving the safe, long-term use of antipsychotic drugs by their patients. Specifically, this book is designed to (1) help inform antipsychotic treatment selections for individual patients (Section 1); and (2) support monitoring of antipsychotic-related side effects over the course of therapy (Sections 2 & 3). For more details, refer to the Guide to using *Antipsychotics and their Side Effects* on p. xx.

Antipsychotics and Their Side Effects was developed as a comprehensive, extensively referenced resource following a semi-systematic approach using three main sources of information: (1) the best available evidence; (2) identification of best practices; and (3) incorporation of our clinical and expert opinion.

Development

There is little or no research that directly assesses the best methods for the monitoring of antipsychotic treatment tolerance or safety. However, selected research and information on the effectiveness, tolerability, and safety of antipsychotics can be used to develop appropriate monitoring practices. Extensive effort was made to locate and review this information. Aided by our research assistants, we conducted searches and literature reviews. Electronic resources used were Medline, EMBASE, the Cochrane Library, PsycINFO, Web of Science, Micromedex Drug Information, and reports from regulatory authorities (e.g. the US Food and Drug Administration, Health Canada). Drug monographs from antipsychotic manufacturers as well as from independent sources (e.g. AHFS Drug Information) along with specialty references (e.g. Meyler's *Side Effects of Drugs* and Joseph and Young's *Movement Disorders in Neurology and Neuropsychiatry*) and health technology assessments were used as appropriate to identify tolerability and safety information. Clinical practice guidelines and published monitoring recommendations were also reviewed. When several studies were identified that addressed the same issue (e.g. diabetes risk with antipsychotic use), the best available evidence as determined by the hierarchy of evidence was selected and used to inform the content.

Limitations

The book offers a unique and clinically valuable resource but is not in itself sufficient for achieving its goals, which are tied directly to the clinician's monitoring practices and systemic supports for monitoring.

Most monitoring recommendations in this book do not derive from studies that were designed to identify the most efficient or effective method for monitoring antipsychotic-related adverse effects. Such studies are effectively non-existent. Rather, the recommendations are a result of several informative components including an assessment of evidence of the risk, frequency, and timing of adverse effects caused by antipsychotics, an assessment of various methods to detect these potential harms, and our clinical judgement.

This guide does not provide information or advice regarding the management of antipsychotic-related adverse effects. The management (or preferably the prevention) of these adverse effects is of critical importance; however, it is beyond the scope of the book. It also does not provide guidance on how to monitor for the desired effects of antipsychotic treatment or what to do if not achieved. For this you are referred to the appropriate clinical practice guideline. This edition also does not specifically review the potential side effects of switching or stopping antipsychotics or how to monitor for them. The information provided applies generally; details related to the side effects and monitoring of antipsychotics when used in unique patient populations, such as the very young and old or during pregnancy and lactation, are not the focus.

The book is intended to supplement good clinical care practice. However, it should not be considered complete in its coverage of potential adverse effects related to antipsychotics or in its recommendations for detecting and monitoring potential adverse effects for all patients. Adjustments or additions to the recommended monitoring may be required for selected patients; for example in pediatric and elderly patients, those on complex drug regimens, or for those with communication limitations. Moreover, application of the information in this guide may not limit or prevent the occurrence of minor or serious adverse effects related to antipsychotics. Users of this book are expected to use their training, knowledge, and judgement regarding the care of their antipsychotic-treated patients in an effort to achieve the desired benefits of treatment while minimizing the treatment-related harms. The guidance offered in this book is not written for non-practitioners.

Guide to using *Antipsychotics and their Side Effects*

This book was developed to support healthcare professionals involved in the care of patients receiving antipsychotic drugs long term. It is hoped that this book will be useful for psychiatrists, family practitioners, nurses, pharmacists, and mental healthcare workers. Some components of the book will also be of benefit to other health professionals, including dieticians and other medical specialists, during their care of patients receiving antipsychotics. Although this book was not developed for patients or their families, they too may find the content useful for making informed treatment decisions and for monitoring guidance.

This book has three major sections, each having a unique clinical utility. Section 1 includes the introduction and 20 concise chapters describing antipsychotic side effects along with the related monitoring recommendations. Each chapter begins with background information about the problem and then provides a summary of the evidence related to specific antipsychotics. General information on how to monitor for the problem, including in some instances how to interpret clinical observations or laboratory results, is provided, followed by an antipsychotic-specific monitoring schedule. Each chapter's monitoring recommendations are consistent in terms of the proposed schedule, and the same symbols are used throughout. These chapters can be used by practitioners to help select an antipsychotic for a specific patient based on the comparative risks for various adverse effects among the different antipsychotics. It also supports practitioners in identifying reasonable methods for the monitoring of adverse effects.

For Section 2, we have created individual antipsychotic monitoring monographs, presented in alphabetical order, that provide clear monitoring recommendations for each antipsychotic. Each monitoring monograph is a reorganization of the information found in Section 1 such that practitioners can easily identify what to monitor and when for each individual antipsychotic. This section of the book will be most useful once the practitioner has selected an antipsychotic and wishes to put a monitoring schedule in place.

In Section 3, we have attempted to distill and somewhat simplify the monitoring recommendations from Sections 1 and 2 into a single general monitoring form that covers most antipsychotic side effects included in the book. To do this, we had to make some compromises, as the monitoring requirements of a patient taking one antipsychotic can be quite different from those when taking a different antipsychotic. However,

we recognize that a general, non-specific monitoring schedule is better than no schedule at all. The monitoring form offered should be combined with the monitoring schedule suggested for the specific antipsychotic prescribed (see Section 2). Moreover, and of critical importance, the clinician should use his or her judgement in modifying the monitoring guide to meet the patient's health needs. Upon first reviewing the form, we expect that it may appear demanding and a bit unclear. To help with the latter, we have provided a guide on how to use the form. To address the concern that the monitoring recommendations may be too demanding, we encourage you to try it out for three to five patients and then determine if it is too demanding or not. We hope your ultimate decision about the value of the form will come from experiencing it. If you would like to create copies of this form and/or would like to adapt it to your needs, it can be downloaded at **www.cambridge.org/9780521132084.**

Lists of appendices, figures, tables, and monitoring schedules

List of Appendices

List of Figures

List of Tables

List of Monitoring Schedules

About the authors

Professor David M. Gardner has been working in mental health for over 20 years. He qualified as a pharmacist in 1988 and has dedicated his career, academic and clinical, to improving how medications are used in the treatment of people living with mental illness. He is a Professor of Psychiatry within the Department of Psychiatry and holds a cross-appointment with the College of Pharmacy of Dalhousie University in Halifax, Nova Scotia, Canada. He mixes teaching and research with his clinical work in the Early Psychosis Program of Nova Scotia. In addition to teaching the therapeutics of psychiatric disorders to various students, practitioners, and patient and family groups, he is well known for his coursework and teachings in how to critically appraise and apply clinical research in practice. Professor Gardner has been recognized for his teaching effectiveness several times by his students and nationally by his peers and he has been an active researcher and publisher in the fields of psychopharmacology and critical appraisal. He is a member of the Science Advisory Committee of the federal Mental Health Commission of Canada whose mandate is to help bring into being an integrated mental health system in Canada that places people living with mental illness at its center.

Dr. Michael D. Teehan is a graduate of the Royal College of Surgeons in Dublin, Ireland. He undertook additional training in Internal Medicine and became a Member of the College of Physicians of Ireland (MRCPI) in 1981, and, by election, was made a Fellow of the College of Physicians of Ireland in 1996. His postgraduate training in Psychiatry began at Trinity College in Dublin, and was completed at Dalhousie University in Halifax, Nova Scotia, Canada. He obtained specialty qualifications (MRCPsych, 1983, and FRCPC,

1984) and has been a member of the active staff of the teaching hospitals in Halifax since that time. His clinical practice, teaching, and research activities have been focused on the severe and persistently mentally ill. More recently, he has worked with the early psychosis population. In addition to direct clinical care, he has been active in the administration of mental health services in the region and province, and has held the position of Clinical Director for Mental Health Services and Psychiatrist in Chief. He was Director of Post-Graduate Training at Dalhousie's Department of Psychiatry from 1994 to 1999, and is currently the Deputy Head in that Department. He was awarded the Community of Scholars Award for Excellence in Clinical Care from the Faculty of Medicine at Dalhousie University in 2002 and the Medical Staff Achievement Award from the Queen Elizabeth Health Sciences Centre in 2003.

About the cover art

Ruthmarie Adams is a self-taught artist and resident of Halifax, Nova Scotia, Canada. She was 26 years of age when she painted this image simply titled *Depression*. It is based on her personal understanding of mental illness. Ruthmarie described the woman in the painting as feeling overwhelmed, lost, and confused. She added, "In the midst of a mental illness the affected person's voice is often not heard. This is symbolized in the painting by the blurred mouth." As a social worker, Ruthmarie supports individuals with mental health challenges to build work skills and the necessary confidence to re-enter the workplace.

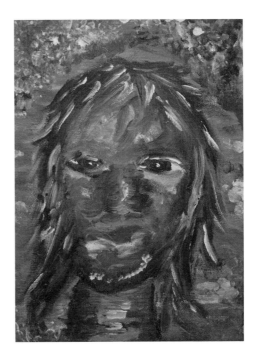

Antipsychotic side effects and monitoring implications

Introduction

A history of side effects

The pharmacological era of dopamine D_2 blockade as the cornerstone of the management of psychoses has its beginnings in the late 1930s with the observation that promethazine, a phenothiazine, prolonged anesthetic sedation. The search for similar agents eventually led to the development of chlorpromazine, which, in the early 1950s, was found to potentiate anesthesia, diminish arousal and locomotion, and produce sleep or indifference, features that eventually came to define the term neuroleptic [1]. Early experience with chlorpromazine in asylums used low doses where it was found to have remarkable calming effects and good tolerability. However, as experience grew and doses increased to 500 mg/day and higher, its remarkable antipsychotic effects became increasingly recognized, bringing a new level of excitement and anticipation to the field of psychiatry [2]. Eventually, clinical experience with chlorpromazine in Europe, Canada, and the USA revealed it to be more than just a calming and sedating agent but also to have ameliorating effects on the cardinal symptoms of psychosis [3]. This started the current era, which is nearing its 60th year, of treating psychosis and mania with dopamine D_2 blockers.

Since the introduction of chlorpromazine, dozens of other antipsychotics have been developed including several other phenothiazines (e.g. thioridazine, mesoridazine, fluphenazine, perphenazine, trifluoperazine), thioxanthenes (e.g. thiothixene, flupenthixol, zuclopenthixol), butyrophenones (e.g. haloperidol), benzepines (e.g. loxapine, clozapine, zotepine) and their structural relatives olanzapine and quetiapine, as well as molindone, pimozide, risperidone and its metabolite paliperidone (9-hydroxyrisperidone), ziprasidone, and aripiprazole. Shortly after its introduction, chlorpromazine was referred to as a "double-edged therapeutic weapon" reflecting its favorable effects in psychoneuroses and psychoses and the early recognition of its frequent and sometimes fatal side effects [4–6]. By 1956, side effects such as sedation, pallor, tachycardia, hypotension, dry mouth, and constipation were well known and almost expected. Serious and fatal cases of pyrexia, skin eruptions, seizures, hepatitis, and agranulocytosis had also been reported. Reversible and irreversible movement disorders were recognized as a class effect shortly thereafter and this had a profound effect on the perception of the safety of neuroleptics [7,8]. Moreover, it gave priority to the importance of routine assessment and monitoring of patients taking antipsychotics long term [9,10].

For approximately 30 years, prescribing an antipsychotic meant using a drug that produced dose-dependent prolactin elevation and extrapyramidal side effects (e.g. parkinsonism, acute dystonia, akathisia) and risked irreversible movement disorders including tardive dyskinesia, dystonia, and akathisia. Prolonged use of high-potency dopamine D_2 blockers (e.g. haloperidol, fluphenazine), especially when used at higher doses, appeared to cause these problems, including neuroleptic malignant syndrome, more often. The alternative of using low-potency agents (e.g. chlorpromazine, thioridazine) carried several additional concerns, including excessive sedation, syncope, hepatitis, cataracts, and seizures [4,5,11]. Over time many prescribers defaulted to the mid-potency agents hoping to find an acceptable compromise (e.g. loxapine), but it was not until clozapine's unique pharmacological and clinical properties were re-assessed and better understood in the late 1980s that new, quite different options were developed in earnest. The return of clozapine in 1989 to the international marketplace provided prescribers and patients with a welcome option of greater effectiveness with little or no risk of movement disorders, of early or late onset, but at the price of higher rates of other serious adverse effects (e.g. agranulocytosis, seizures) [12]. Its greater effectiveness, apparent advantages on negative symptoms and cognitive deficits of schizophrenia, low rate of movement disorders, and unique findings in animal studies were noted to be atypical, and with that a new nomenclature and method of classifying antipsychotics was born. However, when applied to other, newer antipsychotics, the term atypical has been diluted to mean a drug with a lower risk of extrapyramidal side effects and tardive dyskinesia. While every antipsychotic to be marketed since 1990 has been classified as atypical, the term "second generation" seems to be more fitting and carries fewer potentially misleading connotations [1].

The basis of what makes clozapine uniquely effective remains a pharmacological mystery. It has been proposed that its lower risk for movement disorders, along with other second-generation agents, is a result of greater affinity for blocking serotonin (5-hydroxytryptamine, 5-HT_2) receptors compared with dopamine D_2 receptors [13]. Others have found that dopamine D_2 receptor binding properties of antipsychotics, specifically how loosely the drug binds to the receptor as measured by its dissociation constant (K_D), more precisely predict their atypical clinical profile [14]. Antipsychotics with relatively high serotonin 5-HT receptor blocking effects include clozapine, loxapine, olanzapine, paliperidone, quetiapine, risperidone, and ziprasidone [15]. Remoxipride is classified clinically as a second-generation antipsychotic and does not have a high affinity for serotonin receptors, whereas loxapine does but is not considered atypical. Antipsychotics that rapidly dissociate from dopamine D_2 receptors include amoxapine, amisulpride, aripiprazole, clozapine, quetiapine, paliperidone, and remoxipride [16]. Slow to dissociate are chlorpromazine, haloperidol, loxapine, olanzapine, and risperidone. Olanzapine, an extensively prescribed second-generation agent, may owe its lower propensity for parkinsonism to its potent antagonist action at muscarinic receptors. Risperidone is considered to be a dose-dependent second-generation agent, in that it loses its atypical features when dosed above 6 mg/day in adults. Aripiprazole merits special mention as it is the first clinically useful antipsychotic that is not a full antagonist at the dopamine D_2 receptor. Its actions are functionally selective, including antagonist, partial agonist, and agonist, depending on the cell type and function examined [17]. This likely explains its generally low but not absent propensity to cause extrapyramidal and tardive movement effects [18].

New concerns with the second-generation takeover

The development of the second-generation antipsychotics had a profound effect on antipsychotic prescribing. In a few short years, they became not only the agents of choice but also greatly expanded the use of antipsychotics. Off-label use in mood, anxiety, sleep, personality, and impulse control disorders raced ahead of approved new indications by regulators. Across the lifespan, more people today are prescribed antipsychotics than at any time in the past [19–22]. Given this, it comes as no surprise that, in 2008, antipsychotics became the leading revenue generators for their manufacturers, more so than lipid regulators, proton pump inhibitors, and antidepressants [23]. The rapidity of the nearly complete abandonment of the conventional or first-generation antipsychotics is an indicator of the long-standing safety and tolerability concerns with these agents, especially tardive dyskinesia and other potentially irreversible movement disorders. However, the switch has had several consequences, some less foreseeable than others.

Over time, as clinical and research experience with the second-generation antipsychotics accumulated, their negative effects on metabolic and cardiovascular indicators became increasingly obvious. This is particularly unsettling considering that patients for whom antipsychotics are primarily indicated tend to be at much higher risk for obesity, dyslipidemia, hypertension, hyperglycemia, diabetes, and major adverse cardiovascular events such as myocardial infarction, stroke, and sudden cardiac death, and have a markedly reduced expected lifespan, all independent of drug therapy [24–30]. One study estimated that 59% of the excess of deaths in schizophrenia were due to natural causes, led by cardiovascular disease, as compared with 28% due to suicide [31]. Prior to the widespread use of second-generation agents, the risk of dying due to cerebrovascular, cardiovascular, and endocrine causes was found to be two to three times higher in bipolar patients [28]. With schizophrenia, cardiovascular mortality was approximately two times higher, and the rates of ventricular arrhythmias, heart failure, stroke, and diabetes were 1.5 to more than two times that of the general population [29]. It is anticipated that the switch to and expanded use of second-generation antipsychotics will further elevate these risks in adults [32,33].

Although the risk for these prevailing concerns is higher with second- than with first-generation antipsychotics, it should be noted that risk varies within both classes. With the second-generation antipsychotics, clozapine and olanzapine have been identified as most problematic in this regard, while the concerns with risperidone and quetiapine are more moderate, and the more recently introduced ziprasidone and aripiprazole appear to be the safest options, at least in terms of effect on weight and lipids [1,24,34]. Of the first-generation antipsychotics, the low-potency phenothiazines and thioxanthenes are associated with the greatest concerns, while high-potency dopamine D_2 blockers tend to have relatively neutral effects [1,24].

Furthering the concerns about the short- and long-term safety of antipsychotics were the findings of a twofold increased risk in sudden cardiac death across all agents and an increase in overall mortality in elderly patients with dementia [35,36]. A pooled analysis of the safety data collected from 17 randomized controlled trials of second-generation agents in elderly patients with dementia revealed a 60–70% increase in total mortality. At an average follow-up of a mere 10 weeks, the mortality rate with the second-generation antipsychotics was 4.5% compared with 2.6% with placebo. This led to new warnings related to the safety of this class of antipsychotics in the elderly [37]. Several complementary observational studies comparing the risk of death between elderly users of first- and second-generation agents have consistently found that first-generation agents are no safer than the second-generation antipsychotics [38–40]. These findings led regulatory authorities to extend the warnings of increased mortality in the elderly to apply to all antipsychotics [41].

Inadequate medical care for people with mental illness

A positive effect of these new concerns is the enhanced attention and interest given to the overall health of people with chronic psychiatric disorders and to the quality of their healthcare [42]. Quality of care has generally been found to be below that of the general population, especially for people with schizophrenia and substance use disorders. This is a result of several factors related to mental illness, such as greater reluctance to seek or accept medical care and advice, and to service access and delivery [43]. In one study of US veterans with diabetes, the odds of having poor glucose and poor lipid control was increased by 17% and 20%, respectively, in people with mental illness compared with those without, and they were 38% more likely to have had no diabetic monitoring in the previous year [44]. Another study found alarming disparities in the care of patients with mental illness who had experienced an acute myocardial infarction. Compared with people without a mental disorder, they were 20% less likely to be admitted to hospital, 13% less likely to receive reperfusion therapy, and 25% and 32%, respectively, less likely to undergo percutaneous transluminal coronary angioplasty or coronary artery bypass grafting [45]. In a related study, rates of reperfusion and treatment with beta-blockers and angiotensin-converting enzyme (ACE) inhibitors in people with schizophrenia were reduced by 52%, 25%, and 9%, respectively, and 1-year mortality was increased by 34% [46]. Preventive medical services have also been found to be less available to people with major psychiatric disorders [47]. These and other findings have stimulated numerous initiatives to improve the physical healthcare of people with mental illness, including the development of this book.

We were disappointed but not surprised to learn that our patients taking antipsychotics long term, who were known to be at increased risk for metabolic and cardiovascular disease [48], were not being routinely assessed, screened, and monitored for modifiable cardiovascular risk factors. We retrospectively reviewed all outpatient records and emergency visits of 99 randomly selected mental health clinic adult patients to identify what was being monitored and how often. Reflecting the main concerns with contemporary antipsychotic prescribing, and knowing that our patient population is at markedly increased risk for cardiovascular morbidity and mortality, we were primarily interested in weight, body mass index (BMI), waist circumference, smoking status, cholesterol, fasting plasma glucose, blood pressure, and any other evidence of metabolic or cardiovascular disease [49]. To provide some context, we looked for the same information in the outpatient charts of HIV clinic patients at our hospital, another group known to be at higher risk of cardiovascular disease [50]. Based on the information available in the mental health patients' charts, we were able to determine the 10-year coronary artery disease (CAD) risk in only 28% and it took over 2 minutes on average to find this information. In contrast, the better-organized HIV clinic charts had the needed information 90% of the time and it took a mere 18 seconds to find it. We determined that, although our patients are known to be at high risk for diabetes and cardiovascular disease, the importance of this knowledge was not reflected in our

charting practice or charting organization. The sweeping change in prescribing from first-generation antipsychotics, well known for their risk of movement disorders, to second-generation agents, with their high profile metabolic and cardiovascular risks, has not been matched by changes in how patients are being monitored. Change, in this regard, is needed urgently. Our experience is not unique. Evidence of suboptimal screening, assessment, monitoring, and management of the physical health of patients with mental illness is extensive [51–54].

First-generation antipsychotics: down but not out

Concerns regarding the adverse effects of the second-generation antipsychotics on physical health have also stimulated a re-examination of the role of first-generation antipsychotics. Several well-designed non-pharmaceutical industry-sponsored randomized controlled trials and systematic reviews have helped to clarify to what extent the older and newer antipsychotics differ in terms of important clinical outcomes [55–58]. The findings of similar effectiveness, tolerability (although with differing side-effect profiles), and effect on quality of life have supported a modest return of the first-generation agents from the brink of extinction.

Slowly, haltingly, as time goes by, the real facts about any drug emerge into full view [59].

The most recent and most comprehensive systematic review provoked Tyrer and Kendall to comment, "Antipsychotic drugs differ in their potencies and have a wide range of adverse-effect profiles, with nothing that clearly distinguishes the two major groups. Importantly, the second-generation drugs have no special atypical characteristics that separate them from the typical, or first-generation, antipsychotics. As a group they are no more efficacious, do not improve specific symptoms, have no clearly different side-effect profiles than the first-generation antipsychotics, and are less cost effective" [60]. They state that a range of antipsychotics are needed for good clinical practice due to individual variances in response and that all antipsy-chotics are associated in different ways with serious adverse effects that require monitoring. Others have similarly promoted a more balanced approach to the use of first- and second-generation agents than exists today and in doing so advocate increased use of older agents [61]. However, this presents a challenge. For over a decade, the first-generation agents have fallen into disuse. Experienced clinicians have lost some of their skills in treating patients with these agents and newer practitioners have little or no experience with them.

Antipsychotic monitoring in the twenty-first century

Before second-generation antipsychotics were devel-oped, monitoring patients taking antipsychotics required the skills of a neurologist more so than an internist. The focus of monitoring was in the detection of parkinsonism, akathisia, dystonia, and tardive dyskinesia. Several scales were developed to help clinicians reliably detect and measure these drug-induced movement disorders and were standards in the training of psychiatrists and care of patients (e.g. the Simpson Angus Scale for extrapyrami-dal symptoms, the Abnormal Involuntary Movements Scale [AIMS] for tardive dyskinesia, and the comprehen-sive Extrapyramidal Symptom Rating Scale) [62]. Other adverse effect measurement instruments, such as the UKU side-effect rating scale, were developed to assess more comprehensively the side effects of older antipsy-chotics [63].

With the change to second-generation antipsy-chotics, the urgency of monitoring for movement dis-orders quickly diminished and has been replaced by concerns about the development or exacerbation of cardiometabolic risk factors. However, despite numer-ous appeals to improve the medical management of patients taking antipsychotics, a switch in effective, safety-oriented monitoring practices has been slow to evolve [42,54,64]. Several surveys have revealed a per-sistent gap between the awareness of what should be monitored and actual performance [54]. Moreover, it appears that only a small minority of patients are being

monitored according to published recommendations for metabolic and cardiovascular adverse effects, despite acknowledgement that doing so is important and not particularly difficult [49,65-67].

The wide-ranging and consistent findings of inad-equate monitoring practices are not due to a lack of guidance. Several sets of high-profile, widely accessible monitoring recommendations for contemporary anti-psychotic side effects have been available for over 5 years. In early 2004, a joint consensus statement that provided clear guidance on how to monitor for weight gain, dyslipidemia, and diabetes in patients taking anti-psychotics was published by the American Diabetes Association, the American Psychiatric Association, the American Association of Clinical Endocrinologists, and the North American Association for the Study of Obesity [68]. Later in the same year, a broader set of recommendations based on the proceedings of the Mt. Sinai Conference, which was a consensus meeting of psychiatrists and experts in obesity, disease preven-tion, diabetes, cardiology, endocrinology, and ophthal-mology held in October 2002, was also published [64]. Monitoring recommendations covered weight gain, diabetes, dyslipidemia, QT prolongation, hyperprolac-tinemia and sexual dysfunction, extrapyramidal side effects, tardive dyskinesia, cataracts, and myocarditis.

So, what does it take to ensure that patients taking antipsychotics are assessed and monitored appropri-ately? Druss has warned that there is no one-size-fits-all approach to resolving this issue [69]. Instead, he sup-ports the advice from the Institute of Medicine, which encourages the adoption of models that can most easily be built into the existing organizational structure [70]. For clinicians working relatively independently, a change in referral and documentation practices is likely to augment efforts to improve patient monitoring. Referral of patients to primary care services with a clearly articulated request to monitor the patient's physical health can mitigate the burden of doing so alone. For systems with greater opportunity to integrate mental health, primary care, and other medical services, espe-cially when a multidisciplinary approach already exists, there is greater potential for meeting guideline recom-mendations for monitoring and as a result improving patient outcomes [71]. This has been demonstrated in a randomized trial of an integrated model of the primary medical care of patients with severe psychiatric disorders [72]. In this model, improved communications, via phone calls, emails, and in-person meetings, among clinic staff and patients was emphasized and considered critical for success. Even though solutions need to be implemented at the level of the clinician or clinic, health-service administrators and policy makers need to facilitate and support the needed improvements. Without their broad-reaching and enduring support, the many personal efforts, team initiatives, and demonstration projects cannot be expected to have long-lasting effects, especially as they have not done so to date.

Of critical importance for any clinician or health team is to develop standards and processes that ensure systemic assessment, monitoring, and management of potentially reversible medical risk factors, including smoking, dyslipidemia, glucose intolerance, obesity, and hypertension [73]. In parallel, methods of detecting, monitoring, and managing other treatment-related adverse effects, for example movement disorders and hyperprolactinemia-related adverse effects, need to be reviewed and revitalized.

It is also critically important to emphasize the roles of patients and caregivers who are important partners of the monitoring team. This requires effective communication, education, and use of tools to facilitate efficient and accurate assessment of treatment response and tolerability. Patient-oriented education and monitoring tools, such as Med Ed©, which encourages documentation of side effects and treatment response as well as facilitating open communications among patients, caregivers, and members of the treatment team, are simple yet very effective at promoting and supporting effective monitoring [74].

To support the safe and effective use of antipsychotics, especially when used long term, clinicians need to work within a system that supports regular follow-up and monitoring. Establishing a new standard of care in this regard requires planning; personal, professional, and health-team development; effective implementation strategies; and ongoing evaluation. As such, it needs the contribution of effective-change agents and willing clinicians. An integrated, collaborative approach is a must [75].

The change in antipsychotic prescribing preferences and the renewed attention to their adverse effects provides the opportunity for mental health teams to re-examine how they detect and monitor antipsychotic-related adverse effects. Instead of refocusing on the contemporary issues of cardiac and metabolic risk factors, a more comprehensive approach is recommended, one that ensures that patients are being monitored for all potential treatment-related adverse effects [64]. This book was developed to support healthcare practitioners in achieving this goal.

REFERENCES

1. Baldessarini RJ, Tarazi FI. Pharmacotherapy of psychosis and mania. In Brunton LL, Lazo JS, Parker K, eds., *Goodman & Gilman's The Pharmacological Basis of Therapeutics*, 11th edn. New York: McGraw-Hill; 2006.

2. Lambert PA. Chlorpromazine: a true story of the progress effected by this drug. In Ban TA, Healy D, Shorter E, eds., *The Rise of Psychopharmacology and the Story of CINP*. Budapest: Animula; 1998.

3. Swazey JP. *Chlorpromazine in Psychiatry: a Study in Therapeutic Innovation*. Cambridge, MA: MIT Press; 1974.

4. Anonymous. Hazards of chlorpromazine. *Br Med J* 1956;**1** (4963):391–2.

5. Winkelman NW, Jr. Chlorpromazine in the treatment of neuropsychiatric disorders. *J Am Med Assoc* 1954;**155** (1):18–21.

6. Tasker JR Fatal agranulocytosis during treatment with chlorpromazine. *Br Med J* 1955;**1**(4919):950–1.

7. Bockner S. Neurological symptoms with phenothiazines. *Br Med J* 1964;**2**(5413):876.

8. Freyhan FA. Psychomotility and parkinsonism in treatment with neuroleptic drugs. *AMA Arch Neurol Psychiatry* 1957;**78**(5):465–72.

9. Simpson GM, Angus JW. A rating scale for extrapyramidal side effects. *Acta Psychiatr Scand Suppl.* 1970;**212**:11–19.

10. Guy W. *ECDEU Assessment Manual for Psychopharmacology*. Rev. edn. Rockville, MD: U.S. Dept. of Health, Education, and Welfare, Public Health Service, Alcohol, Drug Abuse, and Mental Health Administration, National Institute of Mental Health, Psychopharmacology Research Branch, Division of Extramural Research Programs; 1976.

11. Ayd FJ, Jr. Chlorpromazine: ten years' experience. *JAMA* 1963;**184**:51–4.

12. Baldessarini RJ, Frankenburg FR. Clozapine. A novel antipsychotic agent. *N Engl J Med* 1991;**324**(11):746–54.

13. Meltzer HY, Matsubara S, Lee JC. The ratios of serotonin2 and dopamine2 affinities differentiate atypical and typical antipsychotic drugs. *Psychopharmacol Bull* 1989;**25**(3):390–2.

14. Kapur S, Seeman P. Does fast dissociation from the dopamine D$_2$ receptor explain the action of atypical antipsychotics?: a new hypothesis. *Am J Psychiatry* 2001;**158**(3):360–9.

15. Seeman P. Atypical antipsychotics: mechanism of action. *Can J Psychiatry* 2002;**47**(1):27–38.

16. Seeman P. An update of fast-off dopamine D$_2$ atypical antipsychotics. *Am J Psychiatry* 2005;**162**(10):1984–5.

17. Shapiro DA, Renock S, Arrington E, et al. Aripiprazole, a novel atypical antipsychotic drug with a unique and robust pharmacology. *Neuropsychopharmacology* 2003;**28**(8):1400–11.

18. DeLeon A, Patel NC, Crismon ML. Aripiprazole: a comprehensive review of its pharmacology, clinical efficacy, and tolerability. *Clin Ther* 2004;**26**(5):649–66.

19. Domino ME, Swartz MS. Who are the new users of antipsychotic medications? *Psychiatr Serv* 2008;**59**(5):507–14.

20. Olfson M, Blanco C, Liu L, Moreno C, Laje G. National trends in the outpatient treatment of children and adolescents with antipsychotic drugs. *Arch Gen Psychiatry* 2006;**63**(6):679–85.

21. Mohamed S, Leslie DL, Rosenheck RA. Use of antipsychotics in the treatment of major depressive disorder in the U.S. Department of Veterans Affairs. *J Clin Psychiatry* 2009;**70**(6):906–12.

22. Kamble P, Chen H, Sherer J, Aparasu RR. Antipsychotic drug use among elderly nursing home residents in the United States. *Am J Geriatr Pharmacother* 2008;**6**(4):187–97.

23. IMS Health Incorporated. Top-line industry data: 2008 U.S. sales and prescription information. Top therapeutic classes by U.S. sales. 2008 (cited August 11, 2009). Available from: www.imshealth.com.

24. Gardner DM, Baldessarini RJ, Waraich P. Modern antipsychotic drugs: a critical overview. *CMAJ* 2005;**172**(13):1703–11.

25. Newcomer JW, Hennekens CH. Severe mental illness and risk of cardiovascular disease. *JAMA* 2007;**298**(15):1794–6.

26. Harris EC, Barraclough B. Excess mortality of mental disorder. *Br J Psychiatry* 1998;**173**:11–53.

27. Osby U, Correia N, Brandt L, Ekbom A, Sparen P. Mortality and causes of death in schizophrenia in Stockholm county, Sweden. *Schizophr Res* 2000;**45**(1–2):21–8.

28. Osby U, Brandt L, Correia N, Ekbom A, Sparen P. Excess mortality in bipolar and unipolar disorder in Sweden. *Arch Gen Psychiatry* 2001;**58**(9):844–50.

29. Curkendall SM, Mo J, Glasser DB, Rose Stang M, Jones JK. Cardiovascular disease in patients with schizophrenia in Saskatchewan, Canada. *J Clin Psychiatry* 2004;**65**(5):715–20.

30. Newcomer JW. Medical risk in patients with bipolar disorder and schizophrenia. *J Clin Psychiatry* 2006;**67** Suppl. 9:25–30; discussion 36–42.

31. Brown S. Excess mortality of schizophrenia. A meta-analysis. *Br J Psychiatry* 1997;**171**:502–8.

32. Fontaine KR, Heo M, Harrigan EP, et al. Estimating the consequences of anti-psychotic induced weight gain on health and mortality rate. *Psychiatry Res* 2001;**101**(3):277–88.

33. Casey DE, Haupt DW, Newcomer JW, et al. Antipsychotic-induced weight gain and metabolic abnormalities: implications for increased mortality in patients with schizophrenia. *J Clin Psychiatry* 2004;**65** Suppl. 7:4–18.

34. Newcomer JW. Comparing the safety and efficacy of atypical antipsychotics in psychiatric patients with comorbid medical illnesses. *J Clin Psychiatry* 2009;**70** Suppl. 3:30–6.

35. Ray WA, Chung CP, Murray KT, Hall K, Stein CM. Atypical antipsychotic drugs and the risk of sudden cardiac death. *N Engl J Med* 2009;**360**(3):225–35.

36. Singh S, Wooltorton E. Increased mortality among elderly patients with dementia using atypical antipsychotics. *CMAJ* 2005;**173**(3):252.

37. US Food and Drug Administration. Public health advisory: deaths with antipsychotics in elderly patients with behavioral disturbances. May 7, 2009 (cited August 27, 2009). Available from: http://www.fda.gov/Drugs/DrugSafety/PublicHealthAdvisories/ucm053171.htm.

38. Wang PS, Schneeweiss S, Avorn J, et al. Risk of death in elderly users of conventional vs. atypical antipsychotic medications. *N Engl J Med* 2005;**353**(22):2335–41.

39. Schneeweiss S, Setoguchi S, Brookhart A, Dormuth C, Wang PS. Risk of death associated with the use of conventional versus atypical antipsychotic drugs among elderly patients. *CMAJ* 2007;**176**(5):627–32.

40. Gill SS, Bronskill SE, Normand SL, et al. Antipsychotic drug use and mortality in older adults with dementia. *Ann Intern Med* 2007;**146**(11):775–86.

41. Yan J. FDA extends black-box warning to all antipsychotics. *Psychiatr News* 2008;**43**(14):1.

42. Fleischhacker WW, Cetkovich-Bakmas M, De Hert M, et al. Comorbid somatic illnesses in patients with severe mental disorders: clinical, policy, and research challenges. *J Clin Psychiatry* 2008;**69**(4):514–19.

43. Fagiolini A, Goracci A. The effects of undertreated chronic medical illnesses in patients with severe mental disorders. *J Clin Psychiatry* 2009;**70** Suppl. 3:22–9.

44. Frayne SM, Halanych JH, Miller DR, et al. Disparities in diabetes care: impact of mental illness. *Arch Intern Med* 2005;**165**(22):2631–8.

45. Druss BG, Bradford DW, Rosenheck RA, Radford MJ, Krumholz HM. Mental disorders and use of cardiovascular procedures after myocardial infarction. *JAMA* 2000;**283** (4):506–11.

46. Druss BG, Bradford WD, Rosenheck RA, Radford MJ, Krumholz HM. Quality of medical care and excess mortality in older patients with mental disorders. *Arch Gen Psychiatry* 2001;**58**(6):565–72.

47. Druss BG, Rosenheck RA, Desai MM, Perlin JB. Quality of preventive medical care for patients with mental disorders. *Med Care* 2002;**40**(2):129–36.

48. Kisely S, Smith M, Lawrence D, Cox M, Campbell LA, Maaten S. Inequitable access for mentally ill patients to some medically necessary procedures. *CMAJ* 2007;**176** (6):779–84.

49. Jennex A, Gardner DM. Monitoring and management of metabolic risk factors in outpatients taking antipsychotic drugs: a controlled study. *Can J Psychiatry* 2008;**53** (1):34–42.

50. Bergersen BM, Sandvik L, Bruun JN, Tonstad S. Elevated Framingham risk score in HIV-positive patients on highly active antiretroviral therapy: results from a Norwegian study of 721 subjects. *Eur J Clin Microbiol Infect Dis* 2004;**23**(8):625–30.

51. Morrato EH, Newcomer JW, Kamat S, Baser O, Harnett J, Cuffel B. Metabolic screening after the American Diabetes Association's consensus statement on antipsychotic drugs and diabetes. *Diabetes Care* 2009;**32**(6):1037–42.

52. Himelhoch S, Leith J, Goldberg R, Kreyenbuhl J, Medoff D, Dixon L. Care and management of cardiovascular risk factors among individuals with schizophrenia and type 2 diabetes who smoke. *Gen Hosp Psychiatry* 2009;**31**(1):30–2.

53. Kreyenbuhl J, Medoff DR, Seliger SL, Dixon LB. Use of medications to reduce cardiovascular risk among individuals with psychotic disorders and type 2 diabetes. *Schizophr Res* 2008;**101**(1–3):256–65.

54. Lambert TJ, Newcomer JW. Are the cardiometabolic complications of schizophrenia still neglected? Barriers to care. *Med J Aust* 2009;**190**(4 Suppl.):S39–42.

55. Lieberman JA, Stroup TS, McEvoy JP, et al. Effectiveness of antipsychotic drugs in patients with chronic schizophrenia. *N Engl J Med* 2005;**353**(12):1209–23.

56. Jones PB, Barnes TR, Davies L, et al. Randomized controlled trial of the effect on quality of life of second- vs first-generation antipsychotic drugs in schizophrenia: Cost Utility of the Latest Antipsychotic Drugs in Schizophrenia Study (CUtLASS 1). *Arch Gen Psychiatry* 2006;**63**(10):1079–87.

57. Leucht S, Corves C, Arbter D, Engel RR, Li C, Davis JM. Second-generation versus first-generation antipsychotic drugs for schizophrenia: a meta-analysis. *Lancet* 2009;**373**(9657):31–41.

58. Lewis S, Lieberman J. CATIE and CUtLASS: can we handle the truth? *Br J Psychiatry* 2008;**192**(3):161–3.

59. Dukes MNG. Side effects of drugs essay: the moments of truth. In Dukes MNG, ed., *Side Effects of Drugs Annual*, 1st edn. Amsterdam: Excerpta Medica; 1977.

60. Tyrer P, Kendall T. The spurious advance of antipsychotic drug therapy. *Lancet* 2009;**373**(9657):4–5.

61. Parks J, Radke A, Parker G, et al. Principles of antipsychotic prescribing for policy makers, circa 2008. Translating knowledge to promote individualized treatment. *Schizophr Bull* 2009;**35**(5):931–6.

62. Chouinard G, Ross-Chouinard A, Annable L, Jones B. The extrapyramidal symptom rating scale. *Can J Neurol Sci* 1980;**7**(3):233.

63. Lingjaerde O, Ahlfors UG, Bech P, Dencker SJ, Elgen K. The UKU side effect rating scale. A new comprehensive rating scale for psychotropic drugs and a cross-sectional study of side effects in neuroleptic-treated patients. *Acta Psychiatr Scand Suppl* 1987;**334**:1–100.

64. Marder SR, Essock SM, Miller AL, et al. Physical health monitoring of patients with schizophrenia. *Am J Psychiatry* 2004;**161**(8):1334–49.

65. Feeney L, Mooney M. Atypical antipsychotic monitoring in the Kilkenny mental health services. *Ir J Psychol Med* 2005;**22**(3):101–2.

66. Olson KL, Delate T, Duagn DJ. Monitoring of patients given second-generation antipsychotic agents. *Psychiatr Serv* 2006;**57**(7):1045–6.

67. Nguyen D, Brakoulias V, Boyce P. An evaluation of monitoring practices in patients on second generation antipsychotics. *Australas Psychiatry* 2009;**17**(4):295–9.

68. American Diabetes Association, American Psychiatric Association, American Association of Clinical Endocrinologists, North American Association for the Study of Obesity. Consensus development conference on antipsychotic drugs and obesity and diabetes. *Diabetes Care* 2004;**27** (2):596–601.

69. Druss BG. Improving medical care for persons with serious mental illness: challenges and solutions. *J Clin Psychiatry* 2007;**68** Suppl. 4:40–4.

70. Committee on Crossing the Quality Chasm: Adaptation to Mental Health and Addictive Disorders, Institute of Medicine, Board on Health Care Services. *Improving the Quality of Health Care for Mental and Substance-use Conditions.* Washington, DC: The National Academic Press; 2006.

71. Druss BG, von Esenwein SA. Improving general medical care for persons with mental and addictive disorders: systematic review. *Gen Hosp Psychiatry* 2006;**28**(2):145–53.

72. Druss BG, Rohrbaugh RM, Levinson CM, Rosenheck RA. Integrated medical care for patients with serious psychiatric illness: a randomized trial. *Arch Gen Psychiatry* 2001;**58**(9):861–8.

73. Goff DC, Cather C, Evins AE, et al. Medical morbidity and mortality in schizophrenia: guidelines for psychiatrists. *J Clin Psychiatry* 2005;**66**(2):183–94.

74. Murphy AL, Gardner DM, Kutcher S, Davidson S, Manion I. Collaborating with youth to inform and develop tools for psychotropic decision making. *J Can Acad Child Adolesc Psychiatry* 2010 (in press).

75. Kane JM. Creating a health care team to manage chronic medical illnesses in patients with severe mental illness: the public policy perspective. *J Clin Psychiatry* 2009;**70** Suppl. 3:37–42.

Agranulocytosis and other blood dyscrasias

Background

With the exception of clozapine-induced granulocytopenia and agranulocytosis, most antipsychotic-induced hematological effects are rare and remain poorly characterized. The true incidence of antipsychotic-induced blood dyscrasias has not been estimated accurately.

Antipsychotic agents have been associated with numerous blood dyscrasias, including thrombocytopenia, leukopenia, neutropenia, and agranulocytosis. The mechanism by which antipsychotic agents induce hematological toxicities is currently unknown [1].

Complications of various blood dyscrasias can be severe, even life-threatening. Leukopenia, neutropenia, and agranulocytosis can result in systemic infections and/or death, while profound thrombocytopenia can represent a significant risk of abnormal bleeding.

Agents of interest

Second-generation antipsychotic agents

Aripiprazole

In the premarketing evaluation of aripiprazole, leukopenia, neutropenia, and thrombocytopenia occurred at a rate of between 0.1% and 1% [2].

There is at least one published case of leukopenia associated with aripiprazole and a case of leukopenia and thrombocytopenia associated with the addition of aripiprazole to phenytoin [3,4].

Clozapine

Granulocytopenia and agranulocytosis are well-documented adverse effects associated with clozapine use. The incidence of granulocytopenia is 3%, and the incidence of agranulocytosis is 0.7–0.9%. When agranulocytosis occurs with clozapine, the mortality rate is estimated to be 3–4% [5–7].

The risk of agranulocytosis is much greater with clozapine than with other antipsychotics, including risperidone, olanzapine, quetiapine, and the first-generation agents [8,9].

Age may be a risk factor for developing clozapine-induced agranulocytosis [6].

Roughly 88% of all cases of agranulocytosis occur in the first 6 months of clozapine therapy. A retrospective analysis of 11 555 patients observed a 0.8% risk of agranulocytosis within the first year of clozapine use, and a 0.91% event rate within the first 1.5 years [5,6,10,11].

Due to the frequency and seriousness of clozapine-induced agranulocytosis, many countries, including Canada, the UK, and the USA, require mandatory participation in a special laboratory monitoring program that requires regular (i.e. weekly, biweekly, and monthly) blood monitoring [10].

Clozapine is also associated with eosinophilia and leukocytosis, although these are not as well studied. Incidence is estimated at 0.2% and 0.6% of clozapine patients, respectively. Other blood dyscrasias include thrombocytopenia, thrombocytosis, and acute leukemia. Systemic lupus erythematosus-like syndrome has also been reported [7,12].

Olanzapine

Olanzapine has been implicated in several cases of agranulocytosis. Most occurred within 1 month of starting therapy. Olanzapine, like the other antipsychotics, is safer than clozapine with regard to agranulocytosis risk [13–15].

Several cases of olanzapine-associated neutropenia and leukopenia have been reported; however, the true incidence is unknown [15–19].

There has been at least one case report of thrombocytopenia associated with olanzapine use [20].

Quetiapine

There have been case reports of leukopenia and neutropenia associated with quetiapine use [15,21,22].

Risperidone

There have been isolated reports of leukopenia, neutropenia, and agranulocytosis associated with risperidone [15,23,24].

Ziprasidone

Based on premarketing data, the risk of leucopenia with ziprasidone is estimated to be between 0.1% and 1.0%. Thrombocytopenia risk is rare (<1 per 1000 patients) [25].

There is at least one published case of severe neutropenia associated with ziprasidone [26].

First-generation antipsychotic agents

Phenothiazines

Transient leukopenia is a commonly observed blood test abnormality associated with phenothiazines (e.g. chlorpromazine, perphenazine, thioridazine), with an incidence of approximately one case per three patients. In some, the response is dose-related. White blood cell count reductions are usually mild and transient, with the leukocyte count returning to normal with continued therapy [27,28].

Agranulocytosis has also been reported with phenothiazine therapy. It appears to occur more often in women, and 90% of cases are detected within the first 8 weeks of therapy. The incidence is rare, with imprecise estimates ranging from 1 to 300 per 100 000 patients [9,27,28].

Thioxanthenes

Thiothixene has been implicated in isolated cases of leukopenia, leukocytosis, and neutropenia [27,29].

Haloperidol

There have been reports of mild and usually transient cases of leukopenia and leukocytosis in patients being treated with haloperidol [27,30].

Agranulocytosis has occurred rarely, and only with haloperidol in combination with other medications [27,30].

Other first-generation antipsychotics

There are several reports of transient leukopenia and leukocytosis associated with molindone use [31].

Isolated cases of leukopenia and leukocytosis associated with loxapine therapy have also been reported [32].

Monitoring

Risk factors

There are no clear risk factors associated with antipsychotic-induced blood dyscrasias, although some data suggest age to be a risk factor for clozapine-induced agranulocytosis [6].

Parameters

Blood component	Normal range [33]
Hgb	M: 8.4–10.9 mmol/l (13.5–17.5 g/dl)
	F: 7.4–9.9 mmol/l (12.0–16.0 g/dl)
WBC	$4.5–11.0 \times 10^9$/l
Plt	$150–350 \times 10^9$/l

Hgb = hemoglobin; Plt = platelets; WBC = white blood cell count.

Definitions

	Clinically significant cut-off	Possible signs/symptoms
Agranulocytosis	Granulocyte count $<0.5 \times 10^9$cells/l	Lethargy, weakness, fever, sore throat, flu-like complaints, other signs/symptoms of infection
Neutropenia	ANC $<1.0 \times 10^9$cells/l	
Leukopenia	WBC $<4.0 \times 10^9$cells/l	
Thrombocytopenia	Plt $<150 \times 10^9$cells/l	Impaired clotting presenting as bruising, overt bleeding, melena, decreased Hgb

ANC = absolute neutrophil count; Hgb = hemoglobin; Plt = platelets; WBC = white blood cell count.

Table 1.2.1 Summary of WBC monitoring requirements in the USA and Canada [5,34]

Hematological parameters	Monitoring and treatment implications
USA and Canada:	
WBC $\geq3500/mm^3$ and/or ANC $\geq2000/mm^3$	Continue clozapine and current frequency of monitoring
USA only:	
$3000/mm^3\leq$ WBC $<3500/mm^3$, $1500/mm^3\leq$ ANC $<2000/mm^3$, and/or single drop or cumulative drop within 3 weeks of WBC $\geq3000/mm^3$ or ANC $\geq1500/mm^3$	Monitor twice weekly Continue clozapine
$2000/mm^3\leq$ WBC $<3000/mm^3$ and/or $1000/mm^3\leq$ ANC $<1500/mm^3$	Hold clozapine Monitor daily until WBC $>3000/mm^3$ and ANC $>1500/mm^3$, then twice weekly until WBC $>3500/mm^3$ and ANC $>2000/mm^3$ May rechallenge at this point and monitor weekly for 1 year
WBC $<2000/mm^3$ and/or ANC $<1000/mm^3$	Discontinue treatment and do not rechallenge Monitor until normal and for at least 4 weeks from day of discontinuation
Canada only:	
2.0×10^9/l$\leq$ WBC $<3.5 \times 10^9$/l, or 1.5×10^9/l$\leq$ ANC $<2.0 \times 10^9$/l, or single fall or sum of falls in WBC of $\geq3.0 \times 10^9$/l measured in the last 4 weeks and reaching a value of $<4.0 \times 10^9$/l, or single fall or sum of falls in ANC of $\geq1.5 \times 10^9$/l measured in the last 4 weeks and reaching a value of $<2.5 \times 10^9$/l, or flu-like complaints, fever, or other symptoms suggestive of infection	Monitor twice weekly Continue clozapine
WBC $<2.0 \times 10^9$/l or ANC $<1.5 \times 10^9$/l	Hold clozapine and confirm laboratory results within 24 hours. Stop clozapine if confirmed and do not rechallenge

WBC = white blood cell count; ANC = absolute neutrophil count.

Monitoring schedule for **ANTIPSYCHOTIC-INDUCED AGRANULOCYTOSIS AND OTHER BLOOD DYSCRASIAS**

Monitoring includes complete blood count (CBC) and signs of infection (fever, flu-like complaints, weakness, lethargy, sore throat, etc.)

	Baseline	Weeks		Months					Long-term monitoring
		1	2	1	2	3	6	12	
Second-generation antipsychotics									
Aripiprazole	•								⊛
Clozapine	•	Weekly × 26 weeks, biweekly × 26 weeks, then every 4 weeks thereafter							⊛[a]
Olanzapine	•								⊛
Paliperidone	•								⊛
Quetiapine	•								⊛
Risperidone	•								⊛
Ziprasidone	•								⊛
First-generation antipsychotics									
Chlorpromazine	•								⊛
Flupenthixol	•								⊛
Fluphenazine	•								⊛
Haloperidol	•								⊛
Loxapine	•								⊛
Methotrimeprazine	•								⊛
Molindone	•								⊛
Pericyazine	•								⊛
Perphenazine	•								⊛
Pimozide	•								⊛
Pipotiazine palmitate	•								⊛
Thioridazine	•								⊛
Thiothixene	•								⊛
Trifluoperazine	•								⊛
Zuclopenthixol	•								⊛

• Monitor for adverse effects. ⊛ As clinically indicated.

[a] For clozapine, a CBC with differential reporting of neutrophils is required in Canada, the UK, the USA, and numerous other countries. The requirements of monitoring and reporting vary among regulatory authorities. More intensive monitoring is required when leukocyte counts are reduced. Refer to your local requirements for details. Upon discontinuation of clozapine for any reason, monitoring must be continued for 4 weeks.

Monitoring guidelines

National regulatory bodies vary in their requirements for monitoring. In Canada and the USA during the 1990s and the first few years of the twenty-first century, clozapine was distributed by a single manufacturer (Novartis) and monitoring was carried out by the manufacturer's registry and distribution system. Several parallel monitoring programs now exist in several countries in which clozapine is available as a generic product [5].

In Canada, the UK, and the USA, it is required that blood monitoring of patients taking clozapine occurs weekly for the first 26 weeks of treatment and biweekly for the following 26 weeks. After 1 year of continuous therapy with acceptable hematological results, monitoring may be done every 4 weeks. In Australia, monthly monitoring begins after 6 months of use.

Table 1.2.1 gives a summary of monitoring requirements in the USA and Canada [5,34].

REFERENCES

1. Baldessarini RJ, Tarazi FI. Pharmacotherapy of psychosis and mania. In Brunton LL, Lazo JS, Parker K, eds., *Goodman & Gilman's The Pharmacological Basis of Therapeutics*, 11th edn. New York: McGraw-Hill; 2006.
2. Bristol-Myers Squibb, Otsuka America Pharmaceutical. *Abilify (Aripiprazole) U.S. Full Prescribing Information.* Tokyo, Japan: Otsuka Pharmaceutical Co., Ltd.; 2008.
3. Qureshi SU, Rubin E. Risperidone- and aripiprazole-induced leukopenia: a case report. *Prim Care Companion J Clin Psychiatry* 2008;**10**(6):482–3.
4. Mendhekar D, Duggal H, Andrade C. Leukopenia and thrombocytopenia on adding aripiprazole to phenytoin. *World J Biol Psychiatry* 2008;**7**:1–2.
5. Novartis Pharmaceuticals Canada Inc. *Clozaril (Clozapine) Canadian Prescribing Information.* Dorval, QC: Novartis Pharmaceuticals Canada Inc.; 2007.
6. Alvir JM, Lieberman JA, Safferman AZ, Schwimmer JL, Schaaf JA. Clozapine-induced agranulocytosis. Incidence and risk factors in the United States. *N Engl J Med* 1993;**329**(3):162–7.
7. Iqbal MM, Rahman A, Husain Z, Mahmud SZ, Ryan WG, Feldman JM. Clozapine: a clinical review of adverse effects and management. *Ann Clin Psychiatry* 2003;**15**(1):33–48.
8. Collaborative Working Group on Clinical Trial Evaluations. Adverse effects of the atypical antipsychotics. *J Clin Psychiatry* 1998;**59** Suppl. 12:17–22.
9. Pisciotta V. Drug-induced agranulocytosis. *Drugs* 1978;**15**(2):132–43.
10. Alphs LD, Anand R. Clozapine: the commitment to patient safety. *J Clin Psychiatry* 1999;**60** Suppl. 12:39–42.
11. Patel NC, Dorson PG, Bettinger TL. Sudden late onset of clozapine-induced agranulocytosis. *Ann Pharmacother* 2002;**36**(6):1012–15.
12. Barbui C, Campomori A, Bonati M. Clozapine and blood dyscrasias different from agranulocytosis. *Can J Psychiatry* 1997;**42**(9):981–2.
13. Tolosa-Vilella C, Ruiz-Ripoll A, Mari-Alfonso B, Naval-Sendra E. Olanzapine-induced agranulocytosis: a case report and review of the literature. *Prog Neuropsychopharmacol Biol Psychiatry* 2002;**26**(2):411–14.
14. Naumann R, Felber W, Heilemann H, Reuster T. Olanzapine-induced agranulocytosis. *Lancet* 1999;**354**(9178):566–7.
15. Stergiou V, Bozikas VP, Garyfallos G, Nikolaidis N, Lavrentiadis G, Fokas K. Olanzapine-induced leucopenia and neutropenia. *Prog Neuropsychopharmacol Biol Psychiatry* 2005;**29**(6):992–4.
16. Duggal HS, Gates C, Pathak PC. Olanzapine-induced neutropenia: mechanism and treatment. *J Clin Psychopharmacol* 2004;**24**(2):234–5.
17. Benedetti F, Cavallaro R, Smeraldi E. Olanzapine-induced neutropenia after clozapine-induced neutropenia. *Lancet* 1999;**354**(9178):567.
18. Gajwani P, Tesar GE. Olanzapine-induced neutropenia. *Psychosomatics* 2000;**41**(2):150–1.
19. Kodesh A, Finkel B, Lerner AG, Kretzmer G, Sigal M. Dose-dependent olanzapine-associated leukopenia: three case reports. *Int Clin Psychopharmacol* 2001;**16**(2):117–19.
20. Carrillo JA, Gonzalez JA, Gervasini G, Lopez R, Fernandez MA, Nunez GM. Thrombocytopenia and fatality associated with olanzapine. *Eur J Clin Pharmacol* 2004;**60**(4):295–6.
21. Clark N, Weissberg E, Noel J. Quetiapine and leukopenia. *Am J Psychiatry* 2001;**158**(5):817–18.
22. Cowan C, Oakley C. Leukopenia and neutropenia induced by quetiapine. *Prog Neuropsychopharmacol Biol Psychiatry* 2007;**31**(1):292–4.
23. Finkel B, Lerner AG, Oyffe I, Sigal M. Risperidone-associated agranulocytosis. *Am J Psychiatry* 1998;**155**(6):855–6.
24. Sluys M, Guzelcan Y, Casteelen G, de Haan L. Risperidone-induced leukopenia and neutropenia: a case report. *Eur Psychiatry* 2004;**19**(2):117.

25. Pfizer Canada Inc. *Zeldox (Ziprasidone hydrochloride) Canadian Product Monograph.* Quebec, Canada: Pfizer Canada Inc.; 2007.

26. Montgomery J. Ziprasidone-related agranulocytosis following olanzapine-induced neutropenia. *Gen Hosp Psychiatry* 2006;**28**(1):83–5.

27. American Society of Health-System Pharmacists. Antipsychotics. In McEvoy GK, ed., *AHFS Drug Information.* Bethesda, MD: American Society of Health-System Pharmacists; 2009.

28. Thomson Reuters (Healthcare) Inc. Phenothiazine-induced agranulocytosis and leukopenia. In *DRUGDEX*® *System* (internet database). Greenwood Village, CO: Thomson Reuters (Healthcare) Inc.; 2009 (cited July 9, 2009). Available from: http://www.thomsonhc.com.

29. Thomson Reuters (Healthcare) Inc. Thiothixene. In *DRUGDEX*® *System* (internet database). Greenwood Village, CO: Thomson Reuters (Healthcare) Inc.; 2009 (cited July 9, 2009). Available from: http://www.thomsonhc.com.

30. Thomson Reuters (Healthcare) Inc. Haloperidol. In *DRUGDEX*® *System* (internet database). Greenwood Village, CO: Thomson Reuters (Healthcare) Inc.; 2009 (cited July 9, 2009). Available from: http://www.thomsonhc.com.

31. Thomson Reuters (Healthcare) Inc. Molindone. In *DRUGDEX*® *System* (internet database). Greenwood Village, CO: Thomson Reuters (Healthcare) Inc.; 2009 (cited July 10, 2009). Available from: http://www.thomsonhc.com.

32. Thomson Reuters (Healthcare) Inc. Loxapine. In *DRUGDEX*® *System* (internet database). Greenwood Village, CO: Thomson Reuters (Healthcare) Inc.; 2009 (cited July 10, 2009). Available from: http://www.thomsonhc.com.

33. Kratz A, Ferraro M, Sluss PM, Lewandrowski KB. Case records of the Massachusetts General Hospital. Weekly clinicopathological exercises. Laboratory reference values. *N Engl J Med* 2004;**351**(15):1548–63.

34. Novartis Pharmaceuticals Corporation. *Clozaril (Clozapine) U.S. Prescribing Information.* East Hanover, NJ: Novartis Pharmaceuticals Corporation; 2008.

Anticholinergic effects

Background

Antipsychotic-induced anticholinergic effects occur frequently and result from a blockade of muscarinic receptors (M_1–M_5) in the brain and periphery (Table 1.3.1). In addition to antipsychotics, numerous other commonly used medications have anticholinergic properties (Table 1.3.2).

Common adverse anticholinergic effects include dry mouth, blurred vision, constipation, urinary retention, and cognitive impairment, such as memory difficulties, confusion, and delirium. The cognitive effects caused by anticholinergic medications are especially troublesome in elderly patients. Other less common effects include tachycardia or paradoxical bradycardia, acute closed-angle glaucoma, paralytic ileus, bowel obstruction, psychosis, and sweating impairment with associated hyperthermia [1].

Although anticholinergic effects are often viewed as detrimental, it is important to keep in mind that they can also be beneficial. Anticholinergic medications (such as benztropine) are often used to treat or prevent selected antipsychotic-induced extrapyramidal symptoms (EPS). It should be noted that both desired and undesired anticholinergic effects can result from such treatments [4].

The severity and consequences of a drug's anticholinergic effects are determined by several patient and drug factors. Patient factors include age, comorbid medical conditions (e.g. narrow-angle glaucoma, benign prostatic hypertrophy, urinary retention, dementia, hyperthyroidism, hypertension, congestive heart failure, coronary artery disease), and the concurrent use of other drugs with antimuscarinic effects. Drug factors include dosage, CNS bioavailability, and muscarinic receptor binding affinity (Table 1.3.3) [5].

Agents of interest

Second-generation antipsychotic agents

Aripiprazole

In vitro anticholinergic activity is negligible with aripiprazole at clinically used doses (10–30 mg/day) [9].

In clinical trials, the rates of anticholinergic adverse effects were similar or slightly higher than with placebo [10].

Clozapine

Clozapine is the most anticholinergic of all second-generation antipsychotics. Anticholinergic activity increases with dose [9,11].

Both clozapine and norclozapine plasma levels are strongly correlated with anticholinergic activity, while, among individuals, dose is a relatively poor predictor of anticholinergic effects [11].

Constipation occurs in a dose-dependent manner. In a small trial, frequency of constipation was found to be 0% (0/17) in patients taking 100 mg/day, 16% (4/25) in patients taking 300 mg/day, and 33% (9/27) in patients taking 600 mg/day [11].

There have also been cases of paralytic ileus, an uncommon yet serious side effect, associated with clozapine. In one case, a 42-year-old male

Table 1.3.1 Pharmacological and clinical consequences of muscarinic blockade [1,2]

Organ affected	Pharmacological results of blockade	Possible clinical results of blockade
Eye	Dilation of circular muscle of iris and ciliary muscle, resulting in mydriasis, blockage of aqueous humor outflow, and inability to accommodate	Blurred vision Acute angle closure in patients with narrow-angle glaucoma Falls and impaired activities of daily living
Heart	Sinus tachycardia	Worsening of cardiac or cardiovascular disease (e.g. angina)
Gastrointestinal tract	Depressed gastrointestinal motility	Constipation, paralytic ileus, fecal impaction Nausea, vomiting, bloating, abdominal pain
Oral cavity	Decreased salivary gland secretions	Dry mouth (sialorrhea with clozapine) Decreased nutritional intake Increased risk of infection and cavities Speech difficulties
Urinary tract	Contraction of bladder sphincter and relaxation of bladder wall Inhibition of erection	Urinary retention (especially in men) Incontinence in the elderly Urinary tract infections Sexual dysfunction
Central nervous system	Decreased cholinergic transmission in higher cortical areas Impairment of various executive brain functions	Reduction of extrapyramidal symptoms Memory problems, confusion Agitation, hallucinations, delirium (with higher dosages or in elderly patients) Worsening of dementia

developed postoperative adynamic ileus 7 days after a hemicolectomy. He had been treated with clozapine for 2 years previous to his surgery. In another case, a 30-year-old male developed paralytic ileus following a dose increase of clozapine to 600 mg/day that subsequently resolved when the dose was returned to 450 mg/day. A death has also been reported in association with severe ileus caused by clozapine [12–14].

Clozapine is pharmacologically and clinically more anticholinergic than olanzapine. In an observational study involving 24 patients with schizophrenia, schizoaffective disorder, or bipolar I disorder, the plasma anticholinergic activity of clozapine (444 mg/day) was fivefold higher than olanzapine (15 mg/day). Clozapine-treated patients experienced higher rates of constipation, micturition disturbances, and tachycardia (all $p < 0.05$) but not dry mouth. Sialorrhea was more frequent with clozapine. See Chapter 1.16 for more information regarding antipsychotic-related sialorrhea [15].

Olanzapine

Although olanzapine does produce fewer anticholinergic adverse effects than clozapine, it is considered to be a potent anticholinergic drug. Anticholinergic adverse effects occur in more than 10% of patients [6].

In vitro anticholinergic activity increases in a dose-dependent manner. Olanzapine was found to have higher anticholinergic activity than quetiapine and lower than clozapine [9].

Cases of olanzapine-induced delirium have been documented and are presumed to be related to the drug's anticholinergic activity. One case described a 74-year-old man with dementia who became acutely delirious after 4 days of olanzapine treatment (maximum dose 12.5 mg/day). He was on no other

Table 1.3.2 Medications with moderate or strong anticholinergic activity [3]

Antiarrhythmic	Gastrointestinal/urinary
Disopyramide	antispasmodic – single and
Antiemetic –	combination products containing:
anticholinergic	Belladonna alkaloids
Cyclizine	Atropine
Dimenhydrinate	Hyoscyamine
Meclizine	Scopolamine
Antihistamine	Dicyclomine
Brompheniramine	Flavoxate
Chlorpheniramine	Oxybutynin
Cyproheptadine	Muscle relaxant
Diphenhydramine	Cyclobenzaprine
Doxylamine	Orphenadrine
Hydroxyzine	Selective serotonin reuptake inhibitor
Promethazine	Paroxetine
Triprolidine	Tricyclic antidepressant
Antiparkinsonian-	Amitriptyline
anticholinergic	Clomipramine
Benztropine	Desipramine
Biperiden	Doxepin
Procyclidine	Imipramine
Trihexyphenidyl	Nortriptyline
	Protriptyline
	Trimipramine

Table 1.3.3 Anticholinergic effects and binding affinities of antipsychotics [2,6–8]

Antipsychotic	Clinical anticholinergic effects	Binding affinity[a]
Clozapine	++++	7.5
Thioridazine	++++	10
Chlorpromazine	++++	60
Methotrimeprazine	++++	–
Olanzapine	+++	1.9
Loxapine	++	62.5
Quetiapine	++	120
Fluphenazine	+	2 000
Flupenthixol	+	–
Haloperidol	+	>20 000
Risperidone	+	>10 000

[a] Data are in K_i values (nM): lower numbers indicate higher binding affinity; – indicates data not available. K_i values for individual drugs have been determined in different laboratories; therefore direct comparison is discouraged.

medications. Symptoms resolved within 2 days of stopping olanzapine [16].

Paliperidone

Paliperidone is the active metabolite of risperidone and shares many pharmacological and clinical features, including negligible affinity for muscarinic receptors and placebo rates for anticholinergic adverse effects [17,18].

Quetiapine

Quetiapine has significant affinity for muscarinic receptors, but to a lesser extent than clozapine or olanzapine. *In vitro* anticholinergic activity increases in a dose-dependent fashion [9].

In a meta-analysis comparing quetiapine with placebo, the relative risk (RR) for dry mouth and constipation was 3.7 and 1.9, respectively [19].

Directly comparing the risk of anticholinergic effects between quetiapine and other antipsychotics is difficult due to the confounding effects of variances in dosing schedules used across studies and the concomitant use of anticholinergic drugs to treat extrapyramidal symptoms.

In a 6-week comparison with chlorpromazine (384 mg/day), an antipsychotic with notable anticholinergic effects, quetiapine (407 mg/day) was associated with constipation less frequently (2% vs. 8%) but with similar rates of dry mouth (7.9% vs. 6.0%) and tachycardia (5% vs. 6%) [20].

Risperidone

In vitro anticholinergic activity is negligible with risperidone at clinically used doses (1.5–6 mg/day). Risperidone causes dry mouth less often than olanzapine (RR = 0.50, 95% confidence interval 0.31–0.82) [9,19].

It is unlikely that risperidone causes anticholinergic adverse effects. However, patients taking concomitant anticholinergic drugs to manage risperidone-related EPS can experience them.

Monitoring schedule for **ANTICHOLINERGIC EFFECTS** [a,b]

Monitoring includes assessment of pre-existing, new-onset, and changes in anticholinergic effects, including dry mouth, blurred vision, constipation, urinary retention, and cognitive effects (memory difficulties, confusion, delirium). This is especially important in elderly patients and patients taking other anticholinergic medications.

| | Baseline | Weeks | | Months | | | | | Long-term monitoring |
		1	2	1	2	3	6	12	
Second-generation antipsychotics									
Aripiprazole	•								★
Clozapine	•	•	•	•	•	•	•	•	★
Olanzapine	•			•		•			★
Paliperidone[c]	•	Δ	Δ	Δ	Δ				★
Quetiapine	•			•		•			★
Risperidone[c]	•	Δ	Δ	Δ	Δ				★
Ziprasidone	•								★
First-generation antipsychotics									
Chlorpromazine	•	•	•	•		•			★
Flupenthixol[c]	•	Δ	•	Δ	Δ				★
Fluphenazine[c]	•	Δ	•	Δ	Δ				★
Haloperidol[c]	•	Δ	•	Δ	Δ				★
Loxapine[c]	•	Δ	•	Δ	Δ				★
Methotrimeprazine	•	•	•	•		•			★
Molindone[c]	•	Δ	•	Δ	Δ				★
Pericyazine[c]	•	Δ	•	Δ	Δ				★
Perphenazine[c]	•	Δ	•	Δ	Δ				★
Pimozide[c]	•	Δ	•	Δ	Δ				★
Pipotiazine palmitate[c]	•	Δ	•	Δ	Δ				★
Thioridazine	•	•	•	•		•			★
Thiothixene[c]	•	Δ	•	Δ	Δ				★
Trifluoperazine[c]	•	Δ	•	Δ	Δ				★
Zuclopenthixol[c]	•	Δ	•	Δ	Δ				★

• Monitor for adverse effects. ★ As clinically indicated. Δ Additional monitoring is recommended when an anticholinergic agent is co-prescribed with the antipsychotic.

[a] Anticholinergic effects in patients receiving antipsychotics can be caused by the antipsychotic or by medications used to manage EPS, such as benztropine.

[b] Certain patient populations may require more frequent monitoring for anticholinergic effects, including elderly patients, patients taking other medications with anticholinergic properties, and patients with relevant comorbid medical conditions.

[c] For mid- to high-potency first-generation antipsychotics and high-potency second-generation agents, the regular use of anticholinergic drugs (e.g. benztropine, biperiden, procyclidine) for managing antipsychotic-induced parkinsonism is common. When an anticholinergic is prescribed regularly, monitoring of related side effects is recommended, as indicated.

Ziprasidone

In vitro, ziprasidone demonstrates no anticholinergic activity at clinically used doses (40–160 mg/day) [9].

In a meta-analysis comparing ziprasidone with placebo, the RR for dry mouth was 1.9, but the difference was not statistically significant [19].

First-generation antipsychotic agents

In general, for first-generation antipsychotics, the greatest risk of anticholinergic effects is afforded by agents with low potency at dopamine receptors (e.g. chlorpromazine, methotrimeprazine, thioridazine). There is a low to medium risk of anticholinergic effects associated with medium-potency agents (e.g. perphenazine, thiothixene, loxapine). The risk of anticholinergic effects is very low with high-potency agents (e.g. haloperidol, fluphenazine, trifluoperazine). However, the concurrent use of anticholinergic agents (e.g. benztropine) to manage EPS often produces anticholinergic adverse effects [21].

The first-generation antipsychotics with the greatest anticholinergic effects are thioridazine and chlorpromazine [2].

Monitoring

Prior to initiating antipsychotic therapy, all patients should be assessed for pre-existing anticholinergic effects and risk factors for excessive anticholinergic toxicity. These factors should also be identified throughout the treatment, and therapy should be adjusted accordingly.

In patients with risk factors for severe anticholinergic-related toxicities (e.g. arrhythmias, bowel obstruction, closed-angle glaucoma, dementia, ischemic heart disease, prostatic obstruction), the use of drugs with antimuscarinic effects (e.g. antipsychotics or other agents) should be avoided.

In addition, each time a patient is prescribed a new agent, its potential for inducing anticholinergic effects should be assessed.

REFERENCES

1. Tune LE. Anticholinergic effects of medication in elderly patients. *J Clin Psychiatry* 2001;**62** Suppl. 21: 11–14.

2. Pappano AJ. Cholinoceptor-blocking drugs. In Katzung BG, Masters SB, Trevor AJ, eds., *Basic and Clinical Pharmacology*, 11th edn. New York/London: The McGraw-Hill Companies, Inc.; 2009.

3. Roe CM, Anderson MJ, Spivack B. Use of anticholinergic medications by older adults with dementia. *J Am Geriatr Soc* 2002;**50**(5):836–42.

4. Richelson E. Receptor pharmacology of neuroleptics: relation to clinical effects. *J Clin Psychiatry* 1999;**60** Suppl. 10:5–14.

5. American Society of Health-System Pharmacists. Antimuscarinics/antispasmodics. In McEvoy GK, ed., *AHFS Drug Information*. Bethesda, MD: American Society of Health-System Pharmacists; 2007.

6. Bezchlibnyk-Butler KZ, Jeffries JJ. Antipsychotics (neuroleptics). In Bezchlibnyk-Butler KZ, Jeffries JJ, eds., *Clinical Handbook of Psychotropic Drugs*, 16th edn. Toronto: Hogrefe & Huber Publishers; 2006; p. 77.

7. Gardner DM, Baldessarini RJ, Waraich P. Modern antipsychotic drugs: a critical overview. *CMAJ* 2005 **172** (13):1703–11.

8. Baldessarini RJ, Tarazi FI. Pharmacotherapy of psychosis and mania. In Brunton LL, Lazo JS, Parker K, eds., *Goodman & Gilman's The Pharmacological Basis of Therapeutics*, 11th edn. New York: McGraw-Hill; 2006.

9. Chew ML, Mulsant BH, Pollock BG, et al. A model of anticholinergic activity of atypical antipsychotic medications. *Schizophr Res* 2006;**88**(1–3):63–72.

10. Bristol-Myers Squibb, Otsuka America Pharmaceutical. *Abilify (Aripiprazole) U.S. Full Prescribing Information*. Tokyo, Japan: Otsuka Pharmaceutical Co., Ltd.; 2008.

11. de Leon J, Odom-White A, Josiassen RC, Diaz FJ, Cooper TB, Simpson GM. Serum antimuscarinic activity during clozapine treatment. *J Clin Psychopharmacol* 2003;**23** (4):336–41.

12. Erickson B, Morris DM, Reeve A. Clozapine-associated postoperative ileus: case report and review of the literature. *Arch Gen Psychiatry* 1995;**52**(6):508–9.

13. Rondla S, Crane S. A case of clozapine-induced paralytic ileus. *Emerg Med J* 2007;**24**(2):e12.

14. Hayes G, Gibler B. Clozapine-induced constipation. *Am J Psychiatry* 1995;**152**(2):298.

15. Chengappa KN, Pollock BG, Parepally H, et al. Anticholinergic differences among patients receiving standard clinical doses of olanzapine or clozapine. *J Clin Psychopharmacol* 2000;**20**(3):311–16.

16. Lim CJ, Trevino C, Tampi RR. Can olanzapine cause delirium in the elderly? *Ann Pharmacother* 2006;**40**(1):135–8.

17. Bishara D, Taylor D. Upcoming agents for the treatment of schizophrenia: mechanism of action, efficacy and tolerability. *Drugs* 2008;**68**(16):2269–92.

18. Janssen-Ortho Inc. *Invega (Paliperidone) Canadian Product Monograph.* Toronto, Canada: Janssen-Ortho Inc.; 2008.

19. Bagnall AM, Jones L, Ginnelly L, et al. A systematic review of atypical antipsychotic drugs in schizophrenia. *Health Technol Assess* 2003;**7**(13):1–193.

20. Peuskens J, Link CG. A comparison of quetiapine and chlorpromazine in the treatment of schizophrenia. *Acta Psychiatr Scand* 1997;**96**(4):265–73.

21. Arana GW. An overview of side effects caused by typical antipsychotics. *J Clin Psychiatry* 2000;**61** Suppl. 8:5–11; discussion 12–13.

Diabetes mellitus

Background

Diabetes mellitus is a complex metabolic disorder characterized by elevated dysregulated plasma glucose as a result of a lack of insulin (type 1), insulin insensitivity (type 2), or both. Long term, it is associated with significant morbidity (e.g. myocardial infarction, stroke, infections, amputations, blindness, renal failure, neuropathic pain, erectile dysfunction) and mortality. Acute complications, including diabetic ketoacidosis in type 1 diabetes and hyperglycemic hyperosmolar non-ketotic syndrome in type 2 diabetes, are infrequent but potentially life-threatening and may be the initial presentation of a patient with new-onset diabetes [1,2].

Approximately 15% of people with schizophrenia develop diabetes – a prevalence that is approximately two times greater than the general population [1,3,4].

Schizophrenia is recognized by the Canadian Diabetes Association (CDA) as an independent risk factor for diabetes. The CDA also lists second-generation antipsychotics as a risk factor for diabetes. A joint consensus statement released by the American Diabetes Association, the American Psychiatric Association, the American Association of Clinical Endocrinologists, and the North American Association for the Study of Obesity also recognizes the association between the treatment with second-generation antipsychotics and an increased risk of diabetes [1,4].

People who develop diabetes are categorized as being at high risk for cardiovascular events [1].

Some, but not all, antipsychotic agents have been associated with increases in fasting glucose levels, insulin resistance, glucose intolerance, and the development or unmasking of diabetes [5].

In contrast to some studied antipsychotics (e.g. perphenazine, zuclopenthixol), clozapine and olanzapine are associated with a concentration-dependent increase in circulating insulin levels thought to be secondary to a direct stimulating effect of these agents on pancreatic insulin secretion [6].

Determining causality in the relationship between antipsychotic use and the onset of diabetes can be difficult. People with schizophrenia, who have a significantly higher rate of obesity and metabolic syndrome, are at increased risk for diabetes independent of drug therapy. A baseline assessment of glucose regulation is a requirement if the role of an antipsychotic is to be determined in a case of new-onset diabetes [7,8].

Clinicians managing patients taking antipsychotics long term need to make efforts to prevent diabetes from happening and to detect and respond to it early when it does occur.

Agents of interest

The attributable risk of diabetes associated with antipsychotic use, altogether and for individual agents, has been difficult to assess accurately due to the confounding effect of other prevalent risk factors, variations in the prevalence of these risk factors across studies, inconsistent durations of follow-up, and different case definitions across studies.

Second-generation antipsychotic agents

Aripiprazole

Clinical trial data do not suggest an increased risk of diabetes with aripiprazole; however, there are fewer long-term data for aripiprazole compared with other second-generation agents [4,9].

A large observational study found no increase in risk of being treated for diabetes with aripiprazole (hazard ratio [HR] = 0.93, 95% confidence interval [CI]: 0.50–1.76), quetiapine, risperidone, and ziprasidone, when compared with the rate observed with first-generation antipsychotics. Risk appeared to be increased with clozapine and olanzapine. The cumulative follow-up period was 1323 person-years involving 4528 individuals taking aripiprazole, 16 of whom developed diabetes [10].

Several cases of aripiprazole-associated diabetic emergencies have been reported recently, including a 12-year-old child and three adults who presented with diabetic ketoacidosis and another adult who developed a severe hyperglycemic hyperosmolar non-ketotic coma. Case histories were mixed, with the onset occurring rapidly in some (4 days, 2 weeks) and after extended treatment associated with significant weight gain in others. Type 2 diabetes was known to pre-exist in one case but not in the others [11–15].

Clozapine

Evidence has consistently indicated that clozapine increases the risk of diabetes, possibly more so than any other antipsychotic [10,16–21].

The increase in risk is in addition to the elevated risk of diabetes associated with schizophrenia. Across observational studies, the risk for developing diabetes has been shown consistently to exceed that associated with first-generation antipsychotics, by 25–50% in some studies and higher in others [10,16–20].

An observational study found that clozapine was associated with more than double the rate of new cases of diabetes (HR = 2.58, 95% CI 0.76–8.80) when compared with first-generation antipsychotics. The findings were not statistically significant, possibly due to the small number of cases. The cumulative period of follow-up was only 85 person-years involving 147 clozapine patients of whom three developed diabetes [10].

Significant increases in glucose can occur in as little as 8 weeks of use with clozapine [19].

Phase 2 of the CATIE trial, which randomized 99 phase 1 treatment failures to clozapine, olanzapine, quetiapine, or risperidone, found a mean increase in fasting blood glucose of 9.4 mg/dl (0.5 mmol/l) and a mean increase in glycated hemoglobin (A1C) of 0.11% in clozapine-treated participants over a median follow-up of 9–10 months [22].

Olanzapine

Like clozapine, the evidence linking olanzapine use with an increased risk of glucose intolerance and new-onset diabetes is considerable [16–20,23–27].

The risk of developing diabetes appears to be independent of the risk conferred by schizophrenia and has been demonstrated in multiple comparative observational studies to be greater than the odds of diabetes development attributed to first-generation antipsychotics and risperidone [16–18,23–26].

Significant increases in glucose can occur in as little as 14 weeks [19].

A large observational study found that olanzapine was associated with a 70% higher rate of new-onset diabetes compared with first-generation antipsychotics (HR = 1.71, 95% CI 1.12–2.61). The cumulative period of follow-up was 6745 person-years involving 17 119 olanzapine-treated patients of whom 139 developed diabetes [10].

The CATIE trial (a large, randomized, double-blind, 18-month study that compared olanzapine, perphenazine, quetiapine, risperidone, and ziprasidone in treatment-experienced patients with schizophrenia) showed a mean increase in fasting blood glucose of 13.7 mg/dl (0.8 mmol/l) and a mean increase in A1C of 0.40% in olanzapine-treated participants over a median follow-up of 9 months [27].

Paliperidone

The association between diabetes and paliperidone is not well studied. To date, it has not been included in direct comparison with other agents.

In premarketing clinical trials, there have been few reports of hyperglycemia or other glucose-related events in participants treated with paliperidone [28].

Paliperidone is the active metabolite of risperidone. Its risk of diabetes is not expected to be higher than that observed with risperidone.

Quetiapine

Quetiapine-associated diabetes has been demonstrated in some but not all comparative observational studies to be greater than the risk of diabetes development attributed to first-generation antipsychotics [17,18].

A recent, large observational study found that quetiapine did not increase the risk of diabetes compared with treatment with first-generation antipsychotics (HR = 1.04, 95% CI 0.67–1.62). The cumulative period of follow-up was 6667 person-years involving 17 620 quetiapine patients of whom 89 developed diabetes [10].

Patients treated with quetiapine in the CATIE trial had a mean increase in blood glucose of 7.5 mg/dl (0.4 mmol/l) and in A1C of 0.04%. Relative to the other treatments, its effect on glucose was intermediate and smallest on A1C. However, the median duration of follow-up was 4–5 months, which was shorter than with the other treatments [27].

Risperidone

Risperidone has been associated with the development of glucose intolerance. However, the risk of diabetes is lower compared with clozapine and olanzapine and appears to be on a par with first-generation antipsychotics [16,20,23].

Some studies have found that risperidone does not increase the risk of diabetes (when compared with the risk in untreated patients with schizophrenia) [16–18,23,24].

In the CATIE trial, patients randomized to treatment with risperidone had a mean increase in blood glucose of 6.6 mg/dl (0.4 mmol/l) and in A1C of 0.07% with a median follow-up of about 5 months [27].

The lowest rate of new-onset diabetes was reported with risperidone in a recent, large observational study.

The risk was found to be numerically lower than with first-generation antipsychotics (HR = 0.85, 95% CI 0.54–1.36), although this finding was not statistically significant. The cumulative period of follow-up was 5846 person-years involving 14 838 risperidone patients of whom 57 developed diabetes [10].

Ziprasidone

Compared with other second-generation agents, there are fewer studies describing the risk of glucose abnormalities associated with ziprasidone, but available clinical data suggest little or no increased risk [4].

Treatment with ziprasidone has very rarely been associated with hyperglycemia, exacerbation of pre-existing diabetes, and diabetic coma. However, no causal relationship has been established [29].

Two cases have been published linking new-onset diabetes with ziprasidone treatment [30,31].

A large, observational study showed the risk of new-onset diabetes with ziprasidone to be similar to that observed with first-generation antipsychotics (HR = 1.05, 95% CI 0.54–2.08). The cumulative period of follow-up was 879 person-years involving 2606 ziprasidone patients of whom 13 developed diabetes [10].

In the CATIE trial, patients randomized to treatment with ziprasidone had a mean increase in blood glucose of 2.9 mg/dl (0.2 mmol/l) and in A1C of 0.11% with a median follow-up of about 4 months [27].

First-generation antipsychotic agents

Compared with the data available for the second-generation antipsychotics, there is a paucity of information on the diabetogenic potential of individual first-generation antipsychotic agents.

Studies indicate that first-generation antipsychotics, as a group, may increase the risk of diabetes development by as much as 40% [16,23].

Both high-potency (e.g. haloperidol, fluphenazine) and low-potency (e.g. chlorpromazine, thioridazine) first-generation antipsychotics may have diabetogenic potential [16].

Chlorpromazine

Prospective studies and retrospective analyses from the 1950s–1960s suggest an associated risk of new-onset diabetes with chlorpromazine use [32,33].

Haloperidol

Recent haloperidol-specific data are lacking; however, significant increases in plasma glucose levels have been observed after initiation, although the absolute risk appears small [19].

The risk of new-onset diabetes is reported to be similar to that associated with risperidone [25].

Perphenazine

In the CATIE trial, patients randomized to treatment with perphenazine had a mean increase in blood

Table 1.4.1 Diagnosis of diabetes mellitus [1,2]

Test[a]	Plasma glucose (PG)
Fasting plasma glucose (FPG)	≥126 mg/dl (7.0 mmol/l)
Casual plasma glucose + classic symptoms[b]	≥200 mg/dl (11.1 mmol/l)
Two-hour plasma glucose in a 75 g oral glucose tolerance test	≥200 mg/dl (11.1 mmol/l)

[a] Except for patients presenting with end organ damage characteristic of diabetes mellitus (e.g. nephropathy, neuropathy, retinopathy), a confirmatory test should be scheduled on another day in the absence of unequivocal hyperglycemia accompanied by acute metabolic decompensation.
[b] Classic symptoms of diabetes include polyuria, polydypsia, and unexplained weight loss.

Table 1.4.2 Categories of diagnostic abnormalities in patients at risk of diabetes mellitus

	FPG[a]			Plasma glucose at 2 hours (75 g OGTT)
	ADA	CDA		
IFG	100–125 mg/dl	6.1–6.9 mmol/l		N/A
IFG (isolated)	100–125 mg/dl	6.1–6.9 mmol/l	and	<140 mg/dl (7.8 mmol/l)
IGT (isolated)	<100 mg/dl	<6.1 mmol/l	and	140–199 mg/dl (7.8–11.0 mmol/l)
IFG and IGT	100–125 mg/dl	6.1–6.9 mmol/l	and	140–199 mg/dl (7.8–11.0 mmol/l)

ADA = American Diabetes Association; CDA = Canadian Diabetes Association; FPG = fasting plasma glucose; IFG = impaired fasting glucose; IGT = impaired glucose tolerance; 75 g OGTT = 75 g oral glucose tolerance test; N/A, not applicable.
[a] The ADA and CDA FPG ranges are not identical when converted from imperial to SI units. The ADA has the lower limit for a diagnosis of IFG at an FPG of 100 mg/dl (5.6 mmol/l) with the same upper limit as the CDA at an FPG of 125 mg/dl (6.9 mmol/l).

Table 1.4.3 Glycemic control monitoring parameters for diabetes mellitus [1,2]

	A1C	FPG/preprandial PG	2 hours postprandial PG
Normal range	≤6.0%	ADA: 70–99 mg/dl CDA: 4.0–6.0 mmol/l	ADA: <140 mg/dl CDA: 5.0–8.0 mmol/l
Targets for patients with diabetes	≤7.0%	ADA: 70–130 mg/dl CDA 4.0–7.0 mmol/l	ADA: <180 mg/dl CDA: 5.0–10.0 mmol/l

A1C = glycated hemoglobin; FPG = fasting plasma glucose; PG = plasma glucose; ADA = American Diabetes Association; CDA = Canadian Diabetes Association.

Monitoring schedule for detecting **NEW-ONSET DIABETES**[a]

Monitoring includes a fasting plasma glucose test, preferably, or A1C as well as assessment of signs and symptoms of diabetes. To confirm a diagnosis of diabetes, additional tests may be required if the initial blood test suggests impaired fasting glucose or diabetes.

	Baseline	Weeks 1	Weeks 2	Months 1	Months 2	Months 3	Months 6	Months 12	Long-term monitoring
Untreated	•								★ 12
Second-generation antipsychotics									
Aripiprazole	•						•	•	★ 12
Clozapine	•					•	•	•	★ 6
Olanzapine	•					•	•	•	★ 6
Paliperidone	•						•	•	★ 12
Quetiapine	•						•	•	★ 12
Risperidone	•						•	•	★ 12
Ziprasidone	•						•	•	★ 12
First-generation antipsychotics									
Chlorpromazine	•					•	•	•	★ 6
Flupenthixol	•						•	•	★ 12
Fluphenazine	•						•	•	★ 12
Haloperidol	•						•	•	★ 12
Loxapine	•						•	•	★ 12
Methotrime prazine	•						•	•	★ 12
Molindone	•						•	•	★ 12
Pericyazine	•						•	•	★ 12
Perphenazine	•						•	•	★ 12
Pimozide	•						•	•	★ 12
Pipotiazine palmitate	•						•	•	★ 12
Thioridazine	•						•	•	★ 12
Thiothixene	•						•	•	★ 12
Trifluoperazine	•						•	•	★ 12
Zuclopenthixol	•						•	•	★ 12

• Monitor for adverse effect. ★ As clinically indicated. ⑥ Every 6 months. ⑫ Annually.

[a] For patients with established diabetes, suggested monitoring includes a glycated hemoglobin (A1C) every 3 months and fasting plasma glucose (FPG) at a frequency that varies (e.g. less than daily to multiple daily tests) depending on the situation [1].

glucose of 5.4 mg/dl (3 mmol/l) and in A1C of 0.09% after a median follow-up of 6 months [27].

Monitoring

Risk factors for diabetes mellitus [1]

Age ≥40 years	History of gestational diabetes
First-degree relative with diabetes	History of delivery of a macrosomic infant
Member of high-risk population (e.g. people of Aboriginal, Hispanic, South Asian, Asian, or African descent)	Hypertension Dyslipidemia Overweight
History of impaired glucose tolerance or impaired fasting glucose	Abdominal obesity Polycystic ovary syndrome
Presence of complications associated with diabetes	Acanthosis nigricans Schizophrenia
Vascular disease	Other (refer to [1] for more details)

Table 1.4.1 provides the laboratory criteria for establishing a diagnosis of diabetes based on glucose regulation abnormalities with or without confirmatory clinical findings.

Diagnosis of prediabetes and glucose control targets in diabetes [1,2]

Patients exhibiting glycemic abnormalities described in Table 1.4.2 are at increased risk of developing diabetes. As there are lifestyle and medication interventions that may delay or prevent the progression of diabetes, it is important to identify patients at high risk. The targets of glucose control are provided in Table 1.4.3 in patients with established diabetes.

Useful websites and monitoring tools

• Canadian Diabetes Association 2008 Clinical Practice Guidelines for the Prevention and Management of Diabetes in Canada E-guidelines: http://www.diabetes.ca/for-professionals/resources/2008-cpg/
• Sample Diabetes Patient Care Flow Sheet for Adults (Appendix 2 in CDA 2008 Guidelines, p. S195–6): http://www.diabetes.ca/for-professionals/resources/2008-cpg/

REFERENCES

1. Canadian Diabetes Association Clinical Practice Guidelines Expert Committee. Canadian Diabetes Association 2008 clinical practice guidelines for the prevention and management of diabetes in Canada. *Can J Diabetes* 2008; **32** Suppl. 1:S1–201.
2. American Diabetes Association. Standards of medical care in diabetes – 2009. *Diabetes Care* 2009; **32** Suppl. 1:S13–61.
3. Bushe C, Holt R. Prevalence of diabetes and impaired glucose tolerance in patients with schizophrenia. *Br J Psychiatry Suppl* 2004;**47**:S67–71.
4. American Diabetes Association, American Psychiatric Association, American Association of Clinical Endocrinologists, North American Association for the Study of Obesity. Consensus development conference on antipsychotic drugs and obesity and diabetes. *Diabetes Care* 2004;**27**(2):596–601.
5. Melkersson K, Dahl ML. Adverse metabolic effects associated with atypical antipsychotics: literature review and clinical implications. *Drugs* 2004;**64**(7):701–23.
6. Melkersson KI, Dahl ML, Hulting AL. Guidelines for prevention and treatment of adverse effects of antipsychotic drugs on glucose-insulin homeostasis and lipid metabolism. *Psychopharmacology (Berl)* 2004;**175**(1):1–6.
7. Cohen D, Correll CU. Second-generation antipsychotic-associated diabetes mellitus and diabetic ketoacidosis: mechanisms, predictors, and screening need. *J Clin Psychiatry* 2009;**70**(5):765–6.
8. Stahl SM, Mignon L, Meyer JM. Which comes first: atypical antipsychotic treatment or cardiometabolic risk? *Acta Psychiatr Scand* 2009;**119**(3):171–9.
9. Travis MJ, Burns T, Dursun S, et al. Aripiprazole in schizophrenia: consensus guidelines. *Int J Clin Pract* 2005;**59**(4):485–95.
10. Yood MU, Delorenze G, Quesenberry CP, Jr, et al. The incidence of diabetes in atypical antipsychotic users differs according to agent – results from a multisite epidemiologic study. *Pharmacoepidemiol Drug Saf* 2009;**18**(9):79–9.

11. Church CO, Stevens DL, Fugate SE. Diabetic ketoacidosis associated with aripiprazole. *Diabet Med* 2005;**22**(10):1440–3.

12. Dhamija R, Verma R. Diabetic ketoacidosis induced by aripiprazole in a 12-year-old boy. *Diabetes Care* 2008;**31**(6):e50.

13. Makhzoumi ZH, McLean LP, Lee JH, Ibe AI. Diabetic ketoacidosis associated with aripiprazole. *Pharmacotherapy* 2008;**28**(9):1198–202.

14. Reddymasu S, Bahta E, Levine S, Manas K, Slay LE. Elevated lipase and diabetic ketoacidosis associated with aripiprazole. *JOP* 2006;**7**(3):303–5.

15. Campanella LM, Lartey R, Shih R. Severe hyperglycemic hyperosmolar nonketotic coma in a nondiabetic patient receiving aripiprazole. *Ann Emerg Med* 2009;**53**(2):264–6.

16. Gianfrancesco FD, Grogg AL, Mahmoud RA, Wang RH, Nasrallah HA. Differential effects of risperidone, olanzapine, clozapine, and conventional antipsychotics on type 2 diabetes: findings from a large health plan database. *J Clin Psychiatry* 2002;**63**(10):920–30.

17. Lambert B, Chou CH, Chang KY, Iwamoto T, Tafesse E. Assessing the risk of antipsychotic-induced type II diabetes among schizophrenics: a matched case–control study. *Eur J Neuropsychopharmacology* 2002;**12** Suppl. 3:S307–8.

18. Sernyak MJ, Leslie DL, Alarcon RD, Losonczy MF, Rosenheck R. Association of diabetes mellitus with use of atypical neuroleptics in the treatment of schizophrenia. *Am J Psychiatry* 2002;**159**(4):561–6.

19. Lindenmayer JP, Czobor P, Volavka J, et al. Changes in glucose and cholesterol levels in patients with schizophrenia treated with typical or atypical antipsychotics. *Am J Psychiatry* 2003;**160**(2):290–6.

20. Hedenmalm K, Hagg S, Stahl M, Mortimer O, Spigset O. Glucose intolerance with atypical antipsychotics. *Drug Saf* 2002;**25**(15):1107–16.

21. Smith M, Hopkins D, Peveler RC, Holt RI, Woodward M, Ismail K. First- v. second-generation antipsychotics and risk for diabetes in schizophrenia: systematic review and meta-analysis. *Br J Psychiatry* 2008;**192**(6):406–11.

22. McEvoy JP, Lieberman JA, Stroup TS, et al. Effectiveness of clozapine versus olanzapine, quetiapine, and risperidone in patients with chronic schizophrenia who did not respond to prior atypical antipsychotic treatment. *Am J Psychiatry* 2006;**163**(4):600–10.

23. Koro CE, Fedder DO, L'Italien GJ, et al. Assessment of independent effect of olanzapine and risperidone on risk of diabetes among patients with schizophrenia: population based nested case–control study. *BMJ* 2002;**325**(7358):243.

24. Gianfrancesco F, White R, Wang RH, Nasrallah HA. Antipsychotic-induced type 2 diabetes: evidence from a large health plan database. *J Clin Psychopharmacol* 2003;**23**(4):328–35.

25. Fuller MA, Shermock KM, Secic M, Grogg AL. Comparative study of the development of diabetes mellitus in patients taking risperidone and olanzapine. *Pharmacotherapy* 2003;**23**(8):1037–43.

26. Caro JJ, Ward A, Levinton C, Robinson K. The risk of diabetes during olanzapine use compared with risperidone use: a retrospective database analysis. *J Clin Psychiatry* 2002;**63**(12):1135–9.

27. Lieberman JA, Stroup TS, McEvoy JP, et al. Effectiveness of antipsychotic drugs in patients with chronic schizophrenia. *N Engl J Med* 2005;**353**(12):1209–23.

28. Janssen-Ortho Inc. *Invega (Paliperidone) Canadian Product Monograph.* Toronto, Canada: Janssen-Ortho Inc.; 2009.

29. Pfizer Canada Inc. *Zeldox (Ziprasidone hydrochloride) Canadian Product Monograph.* Quebec, Canada: Pfizer Canada Inc.; 2007.

30. Sanchez-Barranco P. New onset of diabetes mellitus with ziprasidone: a case report. *J Clin Psychiatry* 2005;**66**(2):268–9.

31. Yang SH, McNeely MJ. Rhabdomyolysis, pancreatitis, and hyperglycemia with ziprasidone. *Am J Psychiatry* 2002;**159**(8):1435.

32. Haddad PM. Antipsychotics and diabetes: review of non-prospective data. *Br J Psychiatry Suppl* 2004;**47**:S80–6.

33. Liebzeit KA, Markowitz JS, Caley CF. New onset diabetes and atypical antipsychotics. *Eur Neuropsychopharmacol* 2001;**11**(1):25–32.

Dyslipidemia

Background

Major risk factors for coronary artery disease (CAD) include increasing age, male gender, family history, smoking, hypertension, diabetes, and dyslipidemias (elevated low-density lipoprotein cholesterol [LDL-C] and/or decreased high-density lipoprotein cholesterol [HDL-C]) [1,2].

Patients with schizophrenia and bipolar disorder are more than twice as likely to die from cardiovascular disease compared with the general population [3,4].

Dyslipidemia is defined as serum lipid concentrations outside the desired range. The desired range varies depending on an individual's cardiovascular risk factors [see Tables 1.5.1 and 1.5.2]. There are several different types of lipids. In clinical practice, the most important groups are LDL-C, HDL-C and triglycerides (TGs). It is desirable to keep both serum LDL-C and TGs low, and to keep serum HDL-C high [5,6].

Elevated TG is considered an independent risk factor for CAD; however, its predictive power is not well established [1]. High TG levels are linked with increased cardiovascular risk in people with central obesity, low levels of HDL-C, hypertension and/or insulin resistance. Collectively, when several of these factors present together, it is referred to as metabolic syndrome. According to the American Heart Association and the National Heart, Lung, and Blood Institute, an individual fulfills the criteria for metabolic syndrome when three or more of the following components are present [5,7]:
- Elevated waist circumference:
  - Men: ≥40 inches (102 cm) (for European origin; thresholds vary internationally)
  - Women: ≥35 inches (88 cm) (for European origin; thresholds vary internationally)
- Elevated triglycerides:
  - Equal to or greater than 150 mg/dl
- Reduced HDL ("good") cholesterol:
  - Men: less than 40 mg/dl
  - Women: less than 50 mg/dl
- Elevated blood pressure:
  - Equal to or greater than 130/85 mmHg
- Elevated fasting glucose:
  - Equal to or greater than 100 mg/dl

The ratio of total cholesterol (TC) to HDL-C (TC:HDL-C) is a tool that takes the benefits of elevated HDL relative to the detrimental effects of all other forms of cholesterol into account. TC:HDL-C is considered a more specific predictor of risk compared with measuring TC alone. A low TC:HDL-C ratio is desired [5].

Some, but not all, antipsychotic agents have been associated with dyslipidemia [8–10]. Possible underlying mechanisms include weight gain, dietary changes, and glucose intolerance [11].

Agents of interest

Differences in research methodologies (e.g. different patient populations, definitions used for dyslipidemia, length of studies, etc.) and the limited number of direct comparison randomized clinical trials with long-term follow-up of changes in lipid levels make it difficult to ascertain the true impact of the wide range of antipsychotic agents on lipid profiles or cardiovascular clinical outcomes.

Second-generation antipsychotic agents

Aripiprazole

Available data on aripiprazole suggest that it has minimal effects on serum lipids [9,12].

In a case–control study assessing the risk of dyslipidemia, aripiprazole did not significantly increase the risk of dyslipidemia (odds ratio [OR] = 1.19, 95% confidence interval [CI] 0.94–1.52) compared with those not taking antipsychotics. This was in contrast to the findings with clozapine, risperidone, quetiapine, olanzapine, and ziprasidone, the latter having the second lowest risk (OR = 1.40; 95% CI 1.19–1.65) [13].

Clozapine

Evidence linking clozapine use with an increased risk of dyslipidemia is significant [9,14,15].

An observational study estimated an odds ratio of 1.8 (95% CI 1.6–2.0) regarding the risk of dyslipidemia with clozapine versus no antipsychotic medication [12].

Clozapine has been reported to increase TG concentrations by as much as 45%. Its effects on HDL-C and LDL-C tend to be modest or less [9,14,15].

Olanzapine

Evidence linking olanzapine use with an increased risk of dyslipidemia is significant [9,10,14,15].

In the CATIE trial (a large, double-blind, 18-month randomized trial that compared olanzapine, risperidone, quetiapine, perphenazine, and ziprasidone therapy in patients that were previously on a variety of antipsychotics), olanzapine was associated with the greatest increases in cholesterol (9.4 ± 2.4 mg/dl, $p < 0.001$) and triglycerides (40.5 ± 8.9 mg/dl, $p < 0.001$) [10].

An increase in the risk of dyslipidemia has been found consistently across studies with olanzapine; however, the magnitude of effect varies widely from an odds ratio of 1.5 to 4.5 when compared with similar patients not taking any antipsychotics [13,16].

One observational study determined that for every 1000 patient-years of olanzapine use, approximately 27 people will develop dyslipidemia [16].

Triglycerides can increase approximately 40–60% from baseline in approximately 1 year of olanzapine use [9,17,18].

Other reported olanzapine dyslipidemias include increases in TC, LDL-C, and the TC:HDL-C ratio, and decreases in HDL concentrations. Changes were in the magnitude of approximately 10–15% [9,17,18].

Paliperidone

Data are limited regarding paliperidone's effects on lipids; however, it is not expected to increase lipid levels beyond those observed with risperidone, its parent compound.

The rate of discontinuation due to changes in TGs, HDL, LDL, and TC measurements was not found to be different from with placebo. However, these findings come from 6-week studies, which are not sufficiently long to evaluate this effect [19].

Quetiapine

Available data suggest that quetiapine has the propensity to elevate serum TG concentrations [9,14,15].

In the CATIE trial, quetiapine had the second highest increases in cholesterol (6.6 ± 2.4 mg/dl) and TGs (21.2 ± 9.2 mg/dl) compared with olanzapine, perphenazine, risperidone, and ziprasidone [10].

In an observational study, treatment with quetiapine was associated with a significant increase in the risk of dyslipidemia when compared with no antipsychotic treatment (OR = 1.52, 95% CI 1.40–1.65) [13].

Risperidone

Risperidone has been associated with an increased risk for dyslipidemia, but not consistently across studies. Its effect on lipids is less than with olanzapine [9,10,15,16].

The CATIE trial (which included patients who were taking a variety of antipsychotics prior to enrollment) showed very little change from baseline in cholesterol (-1.3 ± 2.4 mg/dl) or TGs (-2.4 ± 9.1 mg/dl) with risperidone [10].

In one observational trial, the risk for dyslipidemia was no greater with risperidone than with no antipsychotic exposure or with first-generation antipsychotic use [16].

In another trial, risperidone was associated with a significant increase in the risk of dyslipidemia when compared with no antipsychotic medication (OR = 1.53, 95% CI 1.43–1.64) [13].

Regarding TGs specifically, it has been estimated that risperidone use can increase their concentration by 20% over 1 year [16].

Ziprasidone

Ziprasidone's effect on lipids has been extensively evaluated. It is considered to be weight neutral and appears to have less effect on serum lipids than risperidone [9].

In an observational study, ziprasidone was associated with an increased risk of dyslipidemia (OR = 1.40, 95% CI 1.19–1.65) compared with those not taking antipsychotics [13].

Patients taking ziprasidone in the CATIE trial had mean decreases in cholesterol (−8.2±3.2 mg/dl) and TGs (−16.5±12.2 mg/dl). The improved lipid profile likely reflects the discontinuation of previous antipsychotic treatment that promotes lipid accumulation as opposed to a lipid-lowering effect of ziprasidone [10].

First-generation antipsychotic agents

As a group, first-generation antipsychotic agents are associated with a 40% increase in the risk of developing dyslipidemia compared with no antipsychotic exposure [11].

Butyrophenones (e.g. haloperidol) are considered lipid neutral having little or no effect on TGs or TC concentration [9].

Low-potency phenothiazines (e.g. chlorpromazine and thioridazine) have been associated with hypertriglyceridemia. In an analysis of four randomized controlled trials, approximately 20% of patients' baseline cholesterol increased ≥25% over the course of treatment [9,20].

The increase in risk for developing dyslipidemia in an observational study (OR = 1.26, 95% CI 1.14–1.39) was less than that observed for several second-generation agents compared with no antipsychotic medication [13].

Monitoring [1,5]

To determine a patient's target lipid levels, first calculate his or her 10-year cardiovascular risk category using Table 1.5.1. If your patient has established CAD, cerebrovascular disease, peripheral artery disease, chronic kidney disease, and/or diabetes, they are automatically considered high risk due to their pre-existing comorbidities (Table 1.5.2).

Useful websites and monitoring tools

Guidelines

- National Heart, Lung, and Blood Institute (US Department of Health and Human Services): http://www.nhlbi.nih.gov/guidelines/index.htm
- European Society of Cardiology: http://www.escardio.org/guidelines-surveys/esc-guidelines/Pages/GuidelinesList.aspx
- Canadian Cardiovascular Society:
  - Main guidelines site: http://www.ccs.ca/consensus_conferences/cc_library_e.aspx
  - 2009 dyslipidemia guidelines: http://www.ccs.ca/download/consensus_conference/consensus_conference_archives/2009_Dyslipidemia-Guidelines.pdf

Cardiovascular risk calculators

- The HealthyOntario.com heart disease risk calculator (based on the Framingham heart study): http://www.healthyontario.com/HealthTool3.aspx
- The University of Edinburgh Cardiovascular Risk Calculator. This set of calculators allows for greater variation in what is calculated (e.g. stroke, myocardial infarction, coronary heart disease (CHD), cardiovascular disease (CVD), CHD death, CVD death) and the applicability of the calculations: http://cvrisk.mvm.ed.ac.uk/calculator/calc.asp
- Reynolds Risk Score. This tool calculates heart and stroke risk and in addition to the standard variables includes high-sensitivity C-reactive protein (hsCRP) in the estimate: http://www.reynoldsriskscore.org/

Monitoring schedule for **ANTIPSYCHOTIC-INDUCED DYSLIPIDEMIA**[a]

Monitoring includes assessment of lipid profile (TGs, LDL-C, TC:HDL-C ratio) to identify pre-existing, new-onset or worsening dyslipidemia.

	Baseline	Weeks		Months					Long-term monitoring
		1	2	1	2	3	6	12	
Second-generation antipsychotics									
Aripiprazole	•							•	⭐ ⑫
Clozapine	•					•		•	⭐ ⑫
Olanzapine	•					•		•	⭐ ⑫
Paliperidone	•					•		•	⭐ ⑫
Quetiapine	•					•		•	⭐ ⑫
Risperidone	•					•		•	⭐ ⑫
Ziprasidone	•					•		•	⭐ ⑫
First-generation antipsychotics									
Chlorpromazine	•					•		•	⭐ ⑫
Flupenthixol	•							•	⭐ ⑫
Fluphenazine	•					•		•	⭐ ⑫
Haloperidol	•							•	⭐ ⑫
Loxapine	•							•	⭐ ⑫
Methotrimeprazine	•					•		•	⭐ ⑫
Molindone	•							•	⭐ ⑫
Pericyazine	•					•		•	⭐ ⑫
Perphenazine	•					•		•	⭐ ⑫
Pimozide	•							•	⭐ ⑫
Pipotiazine palmitate	•					•		•	⭐ ⑫
Thioridazine	•					•		•	⭐ ⑫
Thiothixene	•							•	⭐ ⑫
Trifluoperazine	•					•		•	⭐ ⑫
Zuclopenthixol	•							•	⭐ ⑫

• Monitor for adverse effect. ⭐ As clinically indicated. ⑫ Annually.

[a] *Note:* although as a group the first-generation antipsychotic agents are associated with dyslipidemias, butyrophenones are considered lipid neutral, while the phenothiazines are associated with hypertriglyceridemia. Therefore, more frequent monitoring is recommended for patients using phenothiazines.

Table 1.5.1 10-year non-fatal myocardial infarction or coronary death risk calculator [2,21]

Men

Age group (years)	Risk points
20–34	−9
35–39	−4
40–44	0
45–49	3
50–54	6
55–59	8
60–64	10
65–69	11
70–74	12
75–79	13

Total cholesterol (mg/dl [mmol/l])	Age group (years)				
	20–39	40–49	50–59	60–69	70–79
<160 (≤4.14)	0	0	0	0	0
160–199 (4.15–5.19)	4	3	2	1	0
200–239 (5.2–6.19)	7	5	3	1	0
240–279 (6.2–7.2)	9	6	4	2	1
>280 (>7.21)	11	8	5	3	1

Smoker	20–39	40–49	50–59	60–69	70–79
No	0	0	0	0	0
Yes	8	5	3	1	1

HDL-C (mg/dl [mmol/l])	
≥60 (≥1.55)	−1
50–59 (1.30–1.54)	0
40–49 (1.04–1.29)	1
<40 (<1.04)	2

Women

Age group (years)	Risk points
20–34	−7
35–39	−3
40–44	0
45–49	3
50–54	6
55–59	8
60–64	10
65–69	12
70–74	14
75–79	16

Total cholesterol (mg/dl [mmol/l])	Age group (years)				
	20–39	40–49	50–59	60–69	70–79
<160 (≤4.14)	0	0	0	0	0
160–199 (4.15–5.19)	4	3	2	1	1
200–239 (5.2–6.19)	8	6	4	2	1
240–279 (6.2–7.2)	11	8	5	3	2
>280 (>7.21)	13	10	7	4	2

Smoker	20–39	40–49	50–59	60–69	70–79
No	0	0	0	0	0
Yes	9	7	4	2	1

HDL-C (mg/dl [mmol/l])	
≥60 (≥1.55)	−1
50–59 (1.30–1.54)	0
40–49 (1.04–1.29)	1
<40 (<1.04)	2

Table 1.5.1 (cont.)

Men

Age group (years) Systolic blood pressure (mmHg)	Risk points	
	Untreated	Treated
<120	0	0
120–129	0	1
130–139	1	2
140–159	1	2
≥160	2	3

Total risk points	10-year risk (%)
<0	<1
0–4	1
5–6	2
7	3
8	4
9	5
10	6
11	8
12	10
13	12
14	16
15	20
16	25
≥17	≥30

Women

Age group (years) Systolic blood pressure (mmHg)	Risk points	
	Untreated	Treated
<120	0	0
120–129	1	3
130–139	2	4
140–159	3	5
≥160	4	6

Total risk points	10-year risk (%)
<9	1
9–12	1
13–14	2
15	3
16	4
17	5
18	6
19	8
20	11
21	14
22	17
23	22
24	27
≥25	>30

Table 1.5.2 Coronary artery disease risk categories and target lipid levels [1,2,5]

Risk category	LDL-C (mg/dl [mmol/l])	TC:HDL-C	TGs (mg/dl [mmol/l])
High risk (10-year risk of coronary artery disease ≥ 20%, or history of diabetes or any atherosclerotic disease)	<100 (<2.0)	<4.0	<150 (<1.7)
Moderate risk (10-year risk of coronary artery disease 10–19%)	<130 (<3.5)	<5.0	<150 (<1.7)
Low risk (10-year risk of coronary artery disease <10%)	<160 (<5.0)	<6.0	<150 (<1.7)

LDL-C = low-density lipoprotein cholesterol; TC:HDL-C = total cholesterol to high-density lipoprotein cholesterol ratio; TGs = triglycerides.

Patient-oriented information about cardiovascular health

- The American Heart Association: http://www.heart.org/heartorg/
- US National Heart, Lung, and Blood Institute: http://www.nhlbi.nih.gov/
- British Heart Foundation: http://www.bhf.org.uk/

REFERENCES

1. Grundy SM, Pasternak R, Greenland P, Smith S, Jr, Fuster V. Assessment of cardiovascular risk by use of multiple-risk-factor assessment equations: a statement for healthcare professionals from the American Heart Association and the American College of Cardiology. *Circulation* 1999;**100**(13):1481–92.
2. McPherson R, Frohlich J, Fodor G, Genest J, Canadian Cardiovascular Society. Canadian Cardiovascular Society position statement – recommendations for the diagnosis and treatment of dyslipidemia and prevention of cardiovascular disease. *Can J Cardiol* 2006;**22**(11):913–27.
3. Osby U, Correia N, Brandt L, Ekbom A, Sparen P. Mortality and causes of death in schizophrenia in Stockholm county, Sweden. *Schizophr Res* 2000;**45**(1–2):21–8.
4. Osby U, Brandt L, Correia N, Ekbom A, Sparen P. Excess mortality in bipolar and unipolar disorder in Sweden. *Arch Gen Psychiatry* 2001;**58**(9):844–50.
5. Genest J, Frohlich J, Fodor G, McPherson R, Working Group on Hypercholesterolemia and Other Dyslipidemias. Recommendations for the management of dyslipidemia and the prevention of cardiovascular disease: summary of the 2003 update. *CMAJ* 2003;**169**(9):921–4.
6. Grundy SM, Cleeman JI, Merz CN, et al. Implications of recent clinical trials for the National Cholesterol Education Program Adult Treatment Panel III Guidelines. *Circulation* 2004;**110**(2):227–39.
7. Eckel RH, Alberti KG, Grundy SM, Zimmet PZ. The metabolic syndrome. *Lancet* 2010;**375**(9710):181–3.
8. Wirshing DA, Pierre JM, Erhart SM, Boyd JA. Understanding the new and evolving profile of adverse drug effects in schizophrenia. *Psychiatr Clin North Am* 2003;**26**(1):165–90.
9. Meyer JM, Koro CE. The effects of antipsychotic therapy on serum lipids: a comprehensive review. *Schizophr Res* 2004;**70**(1):1–17.
10. Lieberman JA, Stroup TS, McEvoy JP, et al. Effectiveness of antipsychotic drugs in patients with chronic schizophrenia. *N Engl J Med* 2005;**353**(12):1209–23.
11. Koro CE, Meyer JM. Atypical antipsychotic therapy and hyperlipidemia: a review. *Essent Psychopharmacol* 2005;**6**(3):148–57.
12. Travis MJ, Burns T, Dursun S, et al. Aripiprazole in schizophrenia: consensus guidelines. *Int J Clin Pract* 2005;**59**(4):485–95.
13. Olfson M, Marcus SC, Corey-Lisle P, Tuomari AV, Hines P, L'Italien GJ. Hyperlipidemia following treatment with antipsychotic medications. *Am J Psychiatry* 2006;**163**(10):1821–5.
14. Melkersson K, Dahl ML. Adverse metabolic effects associated with atypical antipsychotics: literature review and clinical implications. *Drugs* 2004;**64**(7):701–23.
15. Melkersson KI, Dahl ML, Hulting AL. Guidelines for prevention and treatment of adverse effects of antipsychotic drugs on glucose–insulin homeostasis and lipid metabolism. *Psychopharmacology (Berl)* 2004;**175**(1):1–6.
16. Koro CE, Fedder DO, L'Italien GJ, et al. An assessment of the independent effects of olanzapine and risperidone

exposure on the risk of hyperlipidemia in schizophrenic patients. *Arch Gen Psychiatry* 2002;**59**
(11):1021–6.

17. Meyer JM. A retrospective comparison of weight, lipid, and
glucose changes between risperidone- and olanzapine-
treated inpatients: metabolic outcomes after 1 year. *J Clin
Psychiatry.* 2002;**63**(5):425–33.

18. Wirshing DA, Boyd JA, Meng LR, Ballon JS, Marder SR,
Wirshing WC. The effects of novel antipsychotics on
glucose and lipid levels. *J Clin Psychiatry* 2002;**63**
(10):856–65.

19. Janssen-Ortho Inc. *Invega (Paliperidone) Canadian Product
Monograph.* Toronto, Canada: Janssen-Ortho Inc.; 2009.

20. Clark M, Dubowski K, Colmore J. The effect of chlorpromazine on serum cholesterol in chronic schizophrenic
patients. *Clin Pharmacol Ther* 1970;**11**(6):883–9.

21. Expert Panel on Detection, Evaluation, and Treatment
of High Blood Cholesterol in Adults. Executive
summary of the third report of the National Cholesterol
Education Program (NCEP) expert panel on detection, evaluation, and treatment of high blood cholesterol in adults
(adult treatment panel III). *JAMA* 2001;**285**(19):2486–97.

Extrapyramidal symptoms

Background

Extrapyramidal symptoms (EPS) include parkinsonian symptoms (i.e. rigidity, tremor, and bradykinesia), as well as dystonias and akathisia. Tardive (or late) onset movement disorders are discussed in Chapter 1.18. [1].

Antipsychotic-induced rigidity is often unilateral in milder forms, and can be detected by manually rotating the wrists, elbows, shoulders, ankles, and knees. The examiner can typically detect stiffness indicating an increase in muscle tone or a ratcheting resistance referred to as cogwheel rigidity. It is important that the examiner ensures that the patient allows the extremity being examined to go limp. Neuroleptic malignant syndrome should be considered in cases of severe rigidity that has an onset over hours to days (see Chapter 1.8).

Typical parkinsonian resting tremor, characterized by its high amplitude and low frequency, usually presents in the fingers, hands, jaw, tongue, or lips (i.e. rabbit syndrome). Other non-parkinsonian tremors, such as benign familial tremor, tend to have a faster frequency and lower amplitude. They often coexist with typical parkinsonian symptoms and can have multiple causes (e.g. high doses of antipsychotics, caffeine, noradrenergic antidepressants) [2].

Bradykinesia is characterized by slowed movements, diminished spontaneity, masked facial expression, little to no arm swing when walking, and a rigid and often flexed posture. In more severe cases, drooling and disturbed gait can also be present. Bradykinesia is strongly correlated with subjective complaints of tiredness [2].

Acute dystonias are sustained, repetitive, and patterned muscle spasms resulting in twisting, squeezing, pulling, and often painful posturing. Examples include torticollis (neck muscle spasm), trismus (jaw muscle spasm), blepharospasm (blinking spasm), and oculogyric crisis (fixed upward spasm of the eye muscles). While each can present within hours to days after initiating antipsychotic treatment, frequently recurrent, potentially irreversible tardive forms can occur with chronic antipsychotic use (described in Chapter 1.18) [3].

Akathisia presents as motor restlessness, and is accompanied by a strong subjective feeling of inner psychic restlessness. Rocking, pacing, shifting weight while standing, and an inability to remain seated are commonly observed. Patients often describe feeling very tense and uncomfortable, driven to move, and unable to remain still. The drug-induced mechanism of akathisia is not well understood and may not be directly related to D_2 dopamine receptor blockade. Tardive akathisia is also possible with chronic antipsychotic use [4].

Rabbit syndrome is considered a distinct EPS phenomenon affecting the oral and masticatory muscles. It involves fine, rapid, and rhythmic perioral movements, mostly in the vertical plane. These movements are often associated with a popping sound that is produced by the rapid smacking of one's lips. There is evidence that the syndrome involves features of both parkinsonism and tardive dyskinesia. First-generation antipsychotics are clearly associated with rabbit syndrome with prevalence studies reporting rates ranging from 1.5 to 4.4%. There have been no prevalence studies with second-generation agents; only isolated case reports exist [5,6].

Risk factors for antipsychotic-induced EPS include age (children, adolescents, and elderly patients are at higher risk), female gender, Asian ethnicity, a family history of Parkinson's disease, the presence of mood disorders, and antipsychotic dose and potency [2].

Second-generation antipsychotics demonstrate lower risk of EPS over moderate to high doses of first-generation agents. This difference is reduced or erased when compared with low-potency first-generation agents or when anticholinergic drugs are co-prescribed with mid-to-high potency first-generation agents [7–9].

Agents of interest

In general, EPS liability increases with dopamine D_2 receptor blockade. Among first-generation agents, the highest risk for EPS is observed with high-potency agents such as haloperidol and is lowest with low-potency agents such as chlorpromazine. Among the second-generation agents, the same relationship exists between D_2 potency and EPS. See Table 1.6.1 for a comparison of antipsychotic EPS liability.

EPS has been a standard measure of a drug's tolerability in clinical trials. There is an extensive literature examining the EPS liability of older and newer antipsychotics. Drugs of comparison were often either haloperidol at moderate to high doses or, to a much lesser extent, chlorpromazine or other first-generation agents. A welcome exception is the CATIE randomized controlled trial, which had an extended follow-up period of 18 months and included several contemporary antipsychotics (e.g. olanzapine, perphenazine, quetiapine, risperidone, and ziprasidone). Analyses have been completed of people who were free of EPS and tardive dyskinesia when entering the trial and have found small or no differences in the incidences of these side effects [10].

Second-generation antipsychotic agents

Aripiprazole

Among various short-term placebo-controlled studies of people with schizophrenia, bipolar mania, or

Table 1.6.1 EPS risk among antipsychotic drugs [11]

Antipsychotic	EPS liability
Second-generation agents[a]	
Aripiprazole	+
Clozapine	0 to +
Olanzapine	+
Paliperidone	++
Quetiapine	0 to +
Risperidone	++
Ziprasidone	+
First-generation agents	
Low potency	++
Chlorpromazine	
Methotrimeprazine	
Mid potency	+++
Loxapine	
Perphenazine	
Zuclopenthixol	
High potency	++++
Flupenthixol	
Fluphenazine	
Haloperidol	
Pimozide	
Thiothixene	
Trifluoperazine	

[a] Akathisia is possible with all antipsychotics. The risk for acute dystonia and parkinsonism appears correlated to potency at dopamine D_2 receptors. For affinities, refer to Table 1.13.1 in Chapter 1.13.

depression, the risk for EPS with aripiprazole was increased [12].

In placebo-controlled studies involving adults, the increase in EPS rate (excluding akathisia) reported across studies ranged from 1% to 8% with aripiprazole versus placebo. For akathisia, the increased rate observed ranged from 4% to 14% [12].

Two studies were conducted in adolescents, in which higher rates were observed. In both trials, the rate of EPS (excluding akathisia) with aripiprazole was 25%, compared with 5–7% with placebo. Akathisia rates were 9–10% with aripiprazole compared with 2–5% with placebo [12].

There are three published case reports of rabbit syndrome associated with aripiprazole [6,13,14].

Clozapine

The EPS risk with clozapine is very low, but symptoms may be present transiently as a carryover effect from previous treatment with higher-potency antipsychotic agents.

The risk of patients taking clozapine exhibiting a movement disorder is approximately half that of first-generation antipsychotics [15].

In the limited head-to-head studies of clozapine and other second-generation agents, EPS was observed less frequently with clozapine than with risperidone and olanzapine [16,17].

Clozapine commonly causes drooling (affecting ≥50% of patients), but its mechanism is distinct from the parkinsonian drooling observed with other antipsychotics. Clozapine-induced drooling may result from a unique effect of clozapine on the swallowing reflex. For more information, refer to Chapter 1.16 [18].

There is one case report of clozapine-induced rabbit syndrome in a 34-year-old female. Signs emerged after 7 months of clozapine therapy [6].

Olanzapine

The EPS risk with olanzapine is low, but symptoms may be present transiently as a carryover effect from previous treatment with higher-potency antipsychotic agents.

Tremor and akathisia occur more frequently with olanzapine than with placebo; however, the need for anticholinergic drugs to treat EPS is not different from placebo in clinical trials, possibly explained by olanzapine's potent antimuscarinic effect [19].

In comparative studies with first-generation antipsychotics (mostly haloperidol at moderate to high doses), olanzapine patients experience significantly less EPS and use fewer anticholinergics (~75% reduction) [19].

In a 28-week comparison with risperidone used at higher than usual doses (~7 mg/day), EPS were observed less frequently and the need for anticholinergics was reduced by 40% with olanzapine. However, in an 8-week study using lower doses of risperidone (~5 mg), no differences in EPS were observed [20,21].

In people with no evidence of pre-existing parkinsonism allocated to olanzapine in the CATIE trial, parkinsonism was detected in 35%, and 3.7% discontinued treatment as a result. Twenty-two percent experienced akathisia and 2% stopped treatment because of it [10].

Two published case reports of rabbit syndrome associated with olanzapine are known [6,22].

Quetiapine

The EPS risk with quetiapine is very low, but symptoms may be present transiently as a carryover effect from previous treatment with higher-potency antipsychotic agents.

When compared with placebo, the frequency of EPS and the use of anticholinergic drugs used to manage EPS are not increased by quetiapine. The rate of EPS and the use of anticholinergic drugs were both significantly lower with quetiapine than haloperidol, but only slightly less frequent when compared with chlorpromazine [23].

In a single open-label randomized trial, the rate of clinically significant EPS and pharmacotherapy for EPS were both significantly lower with quetiapine (~250 mg) compared with risperidone (~4 mg/day) [24].

In people with no evidence of pre-existing parkinsonism allocated to quetiapine in the CATIE trial, parkinsonism was detected in 29%, and no patient discontinued treatment due to parkinsonism. Seventeen percent experienced akathisia and 1% stopped treatment because of it. Patients taking quetiapine were the least likely to receive parkinsonism medications in this trial [10].

Only one case report of quetiapine-induced rabbit syndrome is known, while in another case rabbit syndrome resolved when treatment was switched to quetiapine [6,25].

Paliperidone

The EPS risk is moderate and dose dependent with paliperidone.

The rate of EPS at doses of up to 6 mg/day is 10–13% and at 9 and 12 mg/day the rates are 25% and 26%, respectively [26].

Two cases of oculogyric crises have been documented in clinical trials [26].

Risperidone

The EPS risk is moderate and dose dependent with risperidone.

The frequency of EPS and the need for anticholinergics is reduced by ~40% with risperidone compared with first-generation antipsychotics (most studies have used moderate to high doses of haloperidol) [27].

Compared with olanzapine, the risk for akathisia is similar with risperidone, but the frequency of parkinsonism and anticholinergic use are higher, especially with higher risperidone doses [20,21,28].

In people with no evidence of pre-existing parkinsonism allocated to risperidone in the CATIE trial, parkinsonism was detected in 37%, and 1.9% discontinued treatment due to parkinsonism. Twenty-five percent experienced akathisia and 2% stopped treatment because of it. Patients taking risperidone were the most likely to receive parkinsonism medications in this trial [10].

There are eight case reports of risperidone-induced rabbit syndrome [6].

Ziprasidone

The EPS risk is low to moderate and is dose dependent with ziprasidone. In short-term, placebo-controlled studies, the overall rate was 14% compared with 8% with placebo [29].

Akathisia occurs more often with ziprasidone (9–12%) than placebo (6%) [30].

The EPS risk appears to be similar to risperidone and olanzapine [30,31].

In people with no evidence of pre-existing parkinsonism allocated to ziprasidone in the CATIE trial, parkinsonism was detected in 32%, and no patient discontinued treatment due to parkinsonism. Twenty percent experienced akathisia and 3% stopped treatment because of it [10].

Based on clinical trial data, oculogyric crisis is listed as occurring at a rate of $\geq$1% [29].

First-generation antipsychotic agents

EPS risk and severity vary by dopamine D_2 receptor potency and dose among the first-generation antipsychotics. High-potency dopamine D_2 antagonists cause more EPS compared with low-potency agents. In general, the risk for EPS is higher among the first-generation agents when compared with the second-generation antipsychotics.

Chlorpromazine

Chlorpromazine, a low-potency D_2 antagonist, was associated with more EPS compared with clozapine in first-episode psychosis patients, and marginally higher rates were observed in a comparison with quetiapine [23,32].

The rate of EPS was similar between olanzapine (alone) and high doses of chlorpromazine (1200 mg) combined with benztropine in treatment-refractory schizophrenia patients [33].

Haloperidol

The EPS risk is moderate to high and is dose dependent with haloperidol, which is a high-affinity dopamine D_2 antagonist.

When combined with a daily dose of the anticholinergic agent benztropine (1–4 mg), the rate of EPS with haloperidol (11–14 mg) is on a par with olanzapine [9].

In patients with first-episode psychosis, ~50% of patients receiving haloperidol (4 mg) experienced parkinsonism and akathisia. This was higher than with olanzapine (11 mg), which had parkinsonism and akathisia rates of ~25% and ~10%, respectively [34].

There are several case reports of rabbit syndrome associated with haloperidol [6].

Perphenazine

The EPS risk is moderate and dose dependent with perphenazine.

In people with no evidence of pre-existing parkinsonism allocated to perphenazine in the CATIE trial, parkinsonism was detected in 30%. Three percent discontinued treatment due to parkinsonism. Twenty-five percent experienced akathisia and 5% stopped treatment because of it [10].

When all patients are considered – those with and without pre-existing EPS – rates of parkinsonism were similar with perphenazine compared with olanzapine, risperidone, quetiapine, and ziprasidone. However, the treatment discontinuation rate due to EPS was higher with perphenazine (8% vs. 2–4% with the second-generation agents) [31].

Monitoring

Before initiating any antipsychotic agent, it is critical that patients be examined for the presence of abnormal movements and that these findings are documented.

Based on current antipsychotic prescribing practices, it is expected that the risk for EPS is higher with first-generation agents compared with second-generation antipsychotics. Within the second-generation agents, risperidone and its active metabolite paliperidone have the highest risk for EPS. To a lesser extent, EPS can be problematic, especially akathisia, with ziprasidone and olanzapine. Patients treated with first-generation agents, paliperidone, or risperidone long term should be formally assessed for the development of EPS more often than patients taking other second-generation agents.

For patients with pre-existing EPS that are switched to an antipsychotic with lower risk, more frequent monitoring of extrapyramidal signs and symptoms are recommended to determine whether or not the abnormal movements are resolving.

Monitoring tools

The Extrapyramidal Symptom Rating Scale (ESRS) is a comprehensive abnormal movement measurement tool and is recommended for monitoring EPS.

The ESRS can be used simply to help remind clinicians what signs and symptoms to look for and document, or it can be used more rigorously by clinicians to document not only the presence or absence of abnormal movements, but also their severity and rate of change over time.

See the Appendix 1.6.1 for a reproduction of the ESRS.

Summary of what to monitor and when

Extrapyramidal symptom	Timing
Akathisia Bradykinesia Rigidity	Early (week 1) and thereafter
Acute dystonia	Early (week 1)
Tremor	Intermediate (week 3) and thereafter

Appendix 1.6.1

Extrapyramidal Symptom Rating Scale (ESRS, Chouinard ©1979)

Reproduced with permission (G. Chouinard, personal communication, October 21, 2007). For detailed ESRS training instructions, see [35].

Summary of the ESRS examination procedure

1. Patient is asked to remove his shoes (omitted if assessment of lower extremities not required). This can follow step 7 if preferred. The patient is asked to remove anything from his mouth (except dentures). The patient is asked to sit facing the examiner on a chair with no armrests.
2. Complete the questionnaire.

Monitoring schedule for **EXTRAPYRAMIDAL SYMPTOMS (EPS)**

Monitoring includes assessment of pre-existing, new-onset, or changes in severity of EPS (using the ESRS – see Appendix 1.6.1). Assessment should include acute dystonia in the early days of treatment and akathisia, bradykinesia, rigidity, and tremor throughout.

	Baseline	Weeks 1	Weeks 2	Months 1	Months 2	Months 3	Months 6	Months 12	Long-term monitoring
Second-generation antipsychotics									
Aripiprazole	•		•		•	•			★ 12
Clozapine	•				•	•			★ 12
Olanzapine	•		•		•	•	•	•	★ 6
Paliperidone	•	•	•	•	•	•	•	•	★ 6
Quetiapine	•			•		•			★ 12
Risperidone	•	•	•	•	•	•	•	•	★ 6
Ziprasidone	•		•	•		•	•	•	★ 6
First-generation antipsychotics									
Chlorpromazine[a]	•	•	•	•	•	•		•	★ 6
Flupenthixol	•	•	•	•	•	•		•	★ 6
Fluphenazine	•	•	•	•	•	•		•	★ 6
Haloperidol	•	•	•	•	•	•		•	★ 6
Loxapine	•	•	•	•	•	•		•	★ 6
Methotrimeprazine[a]	•	•	•	•	•	•		•	★ 6
Molindone	•	•	•	•	•	•		•	★ 6
Pericyazine	•	•	•	•	•	•		•	★ 6
Perphenazine	•	•	•	•	•	•		•	★ 6
Pimozide	•	•	•	•	•	•		•	★ 6
Pipotiazine palmitate	•	•	•	•	•	•		•	★ 6
Thioridazine[a]	•	•	•	•	•	•		•	★ 6
Thiothixene	•	•	•	•	•	•	•	•	★ 6
Trifluoperazine	•	•	•	•	•	•	•	•	★ 6
Zuclopenthixol	•	•	•	•	•	•	•	•	★ 6

• Monitor for adverse effect. ★ As clinically indicated. ⑥ Every 6 months. ⑫ Annually.

[a] Less frequent monitoring of EPS is generally required when low-potency first-generation agents are used at lower doses.

3. Observe facial expressiveness, speech, and dyskinesia while completing the questionnaire.
4. Patient is asked to extend both arms forward, with palms down and eyes closed.
5. The patient is asked to carry out pronation and supination of both hands as fast as possible, and to perform rapid alternate movements of both wrists. If necessary, the finger–nose–finger test may be done.
6. While the patient sits facing the examiner on a chair with no armrests about 1 foot (approx. 30 cm) from a table with his upper body turned, the patient is asked to copy a spiral with each hand and to write the name of his town, province/state, and country.
7. Patient is asked to walk a distance of 12–15 feet (4–5 m) away from and then back towards the examiner.
8. To test postural stability, the patient is asked to stand erect with eyes open with feet slightly apart (1–2 cm). The examiner gently pushes the patient on four sides (each shoulder, back, and chest) while asking the patient to keep his balance.
9. Carry out the examination of the muscular tonus of the four limbs.

Summation of scores

Patient: _____ Date: _____ Examiner: _____

Subjective assessment					Score
I.	Questionnaire				

Objective assessments					
II.	Examination of parkinsonism and akathisia				
III.	Examination of dystonia				
IV.	Examination of dyskinetic movements				

Clinical global impressions					
V.	Dyskinesia severity				
VI.	Parkinsonism severity				
VII.	Dystonia severity				
VIII.	Akathisia				

In case of doubt please score the lesser severity

I. Parkinsonism, akathisia, dystonia, and dyskinesia: questionnaire

In this questionnaire, take into account the verbal report of the patient on the following: 1) the duration of the symptom during the day; 2) the number of days where the symptom was present during the last week; and, 3) the evaluation of the intensity of the symptom by the patient.

Enquire into the status of each symptom and rate accordingly	Absent	Mild	Moderate	Severe	Score
1. Impression of slowness or weakness, difficulty in carrying out routine tasks	0	1	2	3	__
2. Difficulty walking or with balance	0	1	2	3	__
3. Difficulty swallowing or talking	0	1	2	3	__

Enquire into the status of each symptom and rate accordingly	Absent	Mild	Moderate	Severe	Score
4. Stiffness, stiff posture	0	1	2	3	—
5. Cramps or pains in limbs, back, or neck	0	1	2	3	—
6. Restless, nervous, unable to keep still	0	1	2	3	—
7. Tremors, shaking	0	1	2	3	—
8. Oculogyric crisis, abnormal sustained posture	0	1	2	3	—
9. Increased salivation	0	1	2	3	—
10. Abnormal involuntary movements (dyskinesia) of extremities of trunk	0	1	2	3	—
11. Abnormal involuntary movements (dyskinesia) of tongue, jaw, lips, or face	0	1	2	3	—
12. Dizziness when standing up (especially in the morning)	0	1	2	3	—

II. Parkinsonism and akathisia: examination

Items based on physical examinations for Parkinsonism (items 1 to 5)

1. Tremor

Scoring					Items to be scored	Score
		Occasional	Frequent	Constant or almost so	Right upper limb	—
None	0				Left upper limb	—
Borderline	1				Right lower limb	—
Small amplitude		2	3	4	Left lower limb	—
Moderate amplitude		3	4	5	Head	—
Large amplitude		4	5	6	Tongue	—
					Jaw/chin	—
					Lips	—

2. Bradykinesia

	Score
0. Normal	—
1. Global impression of slowness in movements	
2. Definite slowness in movements	
3. Very mild difficulty in initiating movements	
4. Mild to moderate difficulty in initiating movements	
5. Difficulty in starting/stopping any movement, or freezing on initiating voluntary act	
6. Rare voluntary movement, almost completely immobile	

3. Gait and posture

	Score
0. Normal	—
1. Mild decrease of pendular arm movement	
2. Moderate decrease of pendular arm movement, normal steps	
3. No pendular arm movement, head flexed, steps more or less normal	
4. Stiff posture (neck, back), small step (shuffling gait)	
5. More marked, festination, or freezing on turning	
6. Triple flexion, barely able to walk	

4. Postural stability

	Score
0. Normal	—
1. Hesitation when pushed but no retropulsion	
2. Retropulsion but recovers unaided	
3. Exaggerated retropulsion without falling	
4. Absence of postural response; would fall if not caught by examiner	
5. Unstable while standing, even without pushing	
6. Unable to stand without assistance	

5. Rigidity

	Items to be scored	Score
0. Normal muscle tone	Right upper limb	—
1. Very mild, barely perceptible	Right lower limb	—
2. Mild (some resistance to passive movements)	Left upper limb	—
3. Moderate (definite difficulty to move the limb)	Left lower limb	—
4. Moderately severe (moderate resistance but still easy to move limb)		
5. Severe (marked resistance with definite difficulty to move the limb)		
6. Extremely severe (limb nearly frozen)		

Items based on overall observation during examination for Parkinsonism (items 6 to 8)

6. Expressive automatic movements (facial mask/speech)

	Score
0. Normal	—
1. Very mild decrease in facial expressiveness	
2. Mild decrease in facial expressiveness	
3. Rare spontaneous smile, decreased blinking, voice slightly monotonous	
4. No spontaneous smile, staring gaze, low monotonous speech, mumbling	
5. Marked facial mask, unable to frown, slurred speech	
6. Extremely severe facial mask with unintelligible speech	

7. Akathisia

	Score
0. Absent	—
1. Looks restless, nervous, impatient, uncomfortable	
2. Needs to move at least one extremity	
3. Often needs to move one extremity or to change position	
4. Moves one extremity almost constantly if sitting, or stamps feet while standing	
5. Unable to sit down for more than a short period of time	
6. Moves or walks constantly	

8. Sialorrhea

	Score
0. Absent	—
1. Very mild	
2. Mild	
3. Moderate: impairs speech	
4. Moderately severe	
5. Severe	
6. Extremely severe: drooling	

III. Dystonia: examination and observation

Scoring	Items to be scores	1. Acute torsion dystonia score	2. Non-acute or chronic or tardive dystonia
	Right upper limb	—	—
0. Absent	Left upper limb	—	—
1. Very mild	Right lower limb	—	—
2. Mild	Left lower limb	—	—
3. Moderate	Head	—	—
4. Moderately severe	Tongue	—	—
5. Severe	Jaw/chin	—	—
6. Extremely severe	Lips	—	—
	Eyes	—	—
	Trunk	—	—

IV. Dyskinetic movement: examination

Based on examination and observation

1. Lingual movements (slow lateral or torsion movement of tongue)

	Scoring	Occasional[†]	Frequent[†]	Constant or almost so	Score
None	0				—
Borderline	1				
Clearly present within oral cavity		2	3	4	
With occasional partial protrusion		3	4	5	
With complete protrusion		4	5	6	

2. Jaw movements (lateral movement, chewing, biting, clenching)

	Scoring	Occasional[†]	Frequent[†]	Constant or almost so	Score
None	0				—
Borderline	1				
Clearly present, small amplitude		2	3	4	
Moderate amplitude, but without mouth opening		3	4	5	
Large amplitude, with mouth opening		4	5	6	

3. Bucco-labial movements (puckering, pouting, smacking, etc.)

	Scoring	Occasional†	Frequent‡	Constant or almost so	Score
None	0				—
Borderline	1				
Clearly present, small amplitude		2	3	4	
Moderate amplitude, forward movement of lips		3	4	5	
Large amplitude; marked, noisy smacking of lips		4	5	6	

4. Truncal movements (involuntary rocking, twisting, pelvic gyrations)

	Scoring	Occasional†	Frequent‡	Constant or almost so	Score
None	0				—
Borderline	1				
Clearly present, small amplitude		2	3	4	
Moderate amplitude		3	4	5	
Greater amplitude		4	5	6	

5. Upper extremities (choreoathetoid movements only: arms, wrists, hands, fingers)

	Scoring			Score
	Occasional†	Frequent‡	Constant or almost so	
None	0			—
Borderline	1			
Clearly present, small amplitude, movement of one limb	2	3	4	
Moderate amplitude, movement of one limb or movement of small amplitude involving two limbs	3	4	5	
Greater amplitude, movement involving two limbs	4	5	6	

6. Lower extremities (choreoathetoid movements only: legs, knees, ankles, toes)

	Scoring			Score
	Occasional†	Frequent‡	Constant or almost so	
None	0			—
Borderline	1			
Clearly present, small amplitude, movement of one limb	2	3	4	
Moderate amplitude, movement of one limb or movement of small amplitude involving two limbs	3	4	5	
Greater amplitude, movement involving two limbs	4	5	6	

7. Other involuntary movements (swallowing, irregular respiration, frowning, blinking, grimacing, sighing, etc)

Specify: _____

	Scoring			Score
	Occasional†	Frequent‡	Constant or almost so	
None	0			—
Borderline	1			
Clearly present, small amplitude		2	3	4
Moderate amplitude		3	4	5
Greater amplitude		4	5	6

† When activated or rarely spontaneous.

‡ Frequently spontaneous and present when activated.

Items to be scored	Score	Scoring
V. CLINICAL GLOBAL IMPRESSION OF SEVERITY OF DYSKINESIA Considering your clinical experience, how severe is the dyskinesia at this time?	—	0. Absent 1. Borderline
VI. CLINICAL GLOBAL IMPRESSION OF SEVERITY OF PARKINSONISM Considering your clinical experience, how severe is the parkinsonism at this time?	—	2. Very mild 3. Mild
VII. CLINICAL GLOBAL IMPRESSION OF SEVERITY OF DYSTONIA Considering your clinical experience, how severe is the dystonia at this time?	—	4. Moderate 5. Moderately severe 6. Marked
VIII. CLINICAL GLOBAL IMPRESSION OF SEVERITY OF AKATHISIA Considering your clinical experience, how severe is the akathisia at this time?	—	7. Severe 8. Extremely severe

IX. Stage of parkinsonism

	Score
	—

0. Absent

1. Unilateral involvement only, minimal or no functional impairment (stage I)

2. Bilateral or midline involvement, without impairment of balance (stage II)

3. Mildly to moderately disabling: first signs of impaired righting or postural reflex (unsteadiness as the patient turns or when he is pushed from standing equilibrium with the feet together and eyes closed), patient is physically capable of leading independent life (stage III)

4. Severely disabling: patient is still able to walk and stand unassisted but is markedly incapacitated (stage IV)

5. Confinement to bed or wheelchair (stage V)

REFERENCES

1. Marder SR, Essock SM, Miller AL, et al. Physical health monitoring of patients with schizophrenia. *Am J Psychiatry* 2004;**161**(8):1334–49.

2. Osser DN. Neuroleptic-induced pseudoparkinsonism. In Young RR, Joseph AB, eds., *Movement Disorders in Neurology and Neuropsychiatry*, 3rd edn. Malden, MA: Blackwell Science, Inc.; 1999.

3. Miller LG, Jankovic J. Drug-induced dyskinesia: an overview. In Young RR, Joseph AB, eds., *Movement Disorders in Neurology and Neuropsychiatry*, 3rd edn. Malden, MA: Blackwell Science, Inc.; 1999.

4. Tarsy D. Akathisia. In Young RR, Joseph AB, eds., *Movement Disorders in Neurology and Neuropsychiatry*, 3rd edn. Malden, MA: Blackwell Science, Inc.; 1999.

5. Casey DE. Rabbit syndrome. In Young RR, Joseph AB, eds., *Movement Disorders in Neurology and Neuropsychiatry*, 3rd edn. Malden, MA: Blackwell Science, Inc.; 1999.

6. Catena Dell'osso M, Fagiolini A, Ducci F, Masalehdan A, Ciapparelli A, Frank E. Newer antipsychotics and the rabbit syndrome. *Clin Pract Epidemiol Ment Health* 2007;**3**:6.

7. Leucht S, Pitschel-Walz G, Abraham D, Kissling W. Efficacy and extrapyramidal side-effects of the new antipsychotics olanzapine, quetiapine, risperidone, and sertindole compared to conventional antipsychotics and placebo. A meta-analysis of randomized controlled trials. *Schizophr Res* 1999;**35**(1):51–68.

8. Leucht S, Wahlbeck K, Hamann J, Kissling W. New generation antipsychotics versus low-potency conventional antipsychotics: a systematic review and meta-analysis. *Lancet* 2003;**361**(9369):1581–9.

9. Rosenheck R, Perlick D, Bingham S, et al. Effectiveness and cost of olanzapine and haloperidol in the treatment of schizophrenia: a randomized controlled trial. *JAMA* 2003;**290**(20):2693–702.

10. Miller del D, Caroff SN, Davis SM, et al. Extrapyramidal side-effects of antipsychotics in a randomised trial. *Br J Psychiatry* 2008;**193**(4):279–88.

11. Gardner DM, Baldessarini RJ, Waraich P. Modern antipsychotic drugs: a critical overview. *CMAJ* 2005;**172**(13): 1703–11.

12. Bristol-Myers Squibb, Otsuka America Pharmaceutical. *Abilify (Aripiprazole) U.S. Full Prescribing Information.* Tokyo, Japan: Otsuka Pharmaceutical Co., Ltd.; 2008.

13. Caykoylu A, Ekinci O, Kuloglu M, Deniz O. Aripiprazole-induced rabbit syndrome: a case report. *J Psychopharmacol* 2010;**24**(3):429–31.

14. Gonidakis F, Ploubidis D, Papadimitriou G. Aripiprazole-induced rabbit syndrome in a drug-naive schizophrenic patient. *Schizophr Res* 2008;**103**(1–3):341–2.

15. Essali A, Al-Haj Haasan N, Li C, Rathbone J. Clozapine versus typical neuroleptic medication for schizophrenia. *Cochrane Database Syst Rev* 2009;(1):CD000059.

16. Tuunainen A, Wahlbeck K, Gilbody SM. Newer atypical antipsychotic medication versus clozapine for schizophrenia. *Cochrane Database Syst Rev* 2000;(2): CD000966.

17. Meltzer HY, Alphs L, Green AI, et al. Clozapine treatment for suicidality in schizophrenia: international suicide prevention trial (InterSePT). *Arch Gen Psychiatry* 2003;**60**(1):82–91.

18. Davydov L, Botts SR. Clozapine-induced hypersalivation. *Ann Pharmacother* 2000;**34**(5):662–5.

19. Duggan L, Fenton M, Rathbone J, Dardennes R, El-Dosoky A, Indran S. Olanzapine for schizophrenia. *Cochrane Database Syst Rev* 2005;(2):CD001359.

20. Tran PV, Hamilton SH, Kuntz AJ, et al. Double-blind comparison of olanzapine versus risperidone in the treatment of schizophrenia and other psychotic disorders. *J Clin Psychopharmacol* 1997;**17**(5):407–18.

21. Conley RR, Mahmoud R. A randomized double-blind study of risperidone and olanzapine in the treatment of schizophrenia or schizoaffective disorder. *Am J Psychiatry* 2001;**158**(5):765–74.

22. Praharaj SK, Sarkar S, Jana AK, Sinha VK. Olanzapine-induced rabbit syndrome. *South Med J* 2008;**101**(10): 1069–70.

23. Srisurapanont M, Maneeton B, Maneeton N. Quetiapine for schizophrenia. *Cochrane Database Syst Rev* 2004;(2): CD000967.

24. Mullen J, Jibson MD, Sweitzer D. A comparison of the relative safety, efficacy, and tolerability of quetiapine and risperidone in outpatients with schizophrenia and other psychotic disorders: the quetiapine experience with safety and tolerability (QUEST) study. *Clin Ther* 2001;**23** (11):1839–54.

25. Wu CC, Su KP. Quetiapine-induced rabbit syndrome in a patient with bipolar disorder. *Prog Neuropsychopharmacol Biol Psychiatry* 2008;**32**(8):2002–3.

26. Janssen-Ortho Inc. *Invega (Paliperidone) Canadian Product Monograph.* Toronto, Canada: Janssen-Ortho Inc.; 2009.

27. Hunter RH, Joy CB, Kennedy E, Gilbody SM, Song F. Risperidone versus typical antipsychotic medication for schizophrenia. *Cochrane Database Syst Rev* 2003;(2): CD000440.

28. Gilbody SM, Bagnall AM, Duggan L, Tuunainen A. Risperidone versus other atypical antipsychotic medication for schizophrenia. *Cochrane Database Syst Rev* 2000;(3): CD002306.

29. Pfizer Canada Inc. *Zeldox (Ziprasidone hydrochloride) Canadian Product Monograph.* Quebec, Canada: Pfizer Canada Inc.; 2007.

30. Kutcher S, Brooks SJ, Gardner DM, et al. Expert Canadian consensus suggestions on the rational, clinical use of ziprasidone in the treatment of schizophrenia and related psychotic disorders. *Neuropsychiatr Dis Treat* 2005;**1**(2):89–108.

31. Lieberman JA, Stroup TS, McEvoy JP, et al. Effectiveness of antipsychotic drugs in patients with chronic schizophrenia. *N Engl J Med* 2005;**353**(12):1209–23.

32. Lieberman JA, Phillips M, Gu H, et al. Atypical and conventional antipsychotic drugs in treatment-naive first-episode schizophrenia: a 52-week randomized trial of clozapine vs chlorpromazine. *Neuropsychopharmacology* 2003;**28**(5):995–1003.

33. Conley RR, Tamminga CA, Bartko JJ, et al. Olanzapine compared with chlorpromazine in treatment-resistant schizophrenia. *Am J Psychiatry* 1998;**155**(7):914–20.

34. Lieberman JA, Tollefson G, Tohen M, et al. Comparative efficacy and safety of atypical and conventional antipsychotic drugs in first-episode psychosis: a randomized, double-blind trial of olanzapine versus haloperidol. *Am J Psychiatry* 2003;**160**(8):1396–404.

35. Chouinard G, Margolese HC. Manual for the extrapyramidal symptom rating scale (ESRS). *Schizophr Res* 2005;**76** (2–3):247–65.

Hepatic effects

Background

Drugs are but one of many possible causes of hepatic injury. Others include genetic diseases (such as hemochromatosis and Wilson's disease), gallstones, hepatitis B and C viruses, alcohol, obesity, autoimmune disorders, and malignancy [1,2].

Numerous medications are associated with drug-induced hepatic damage. The risk of serious hepatic injury is rare, unpredictable, and typically not related to dosage. Drug-induced liver damage can be either cholestatic or hepatocellular. Cholestasis involves abnormalities in the metabolism or secretion of bile, and is usually secondary to biliary flow obstruction. Hepatocellular liver damage results from inflamed or damaged hepatocytes [1].

Elevation of hepatic enzymes tends to be transient with antipsychotic drugs. Consequently, when hepatic enzymes are found to be mildly elevated, drug therapy does not need to be interrupted in most cases. Enzyme elevations of two to three times above the upper limit of normal (ULN) do not require drug discontinuation but warrant follow-up monitoring due to the potential risk of liver damage (e.g. fulminant hepatic necrosis) with continued medication exposure. Continuous minor elevations in liver enzymes do not appear to pose a threat to liver function [3–5].

Treatment should be held when enzyme levels exceed three times the ULN (Table 1.17.1) and the cause of the hepatic injury should be investigated to determine whether or not the antipsychotic is causative. Other causes should be considered, especially excessive alcohol and substance use, which are common among patients with schizophrenia and bipolar disorder [6].

Agents of interest

Most information regarding the potential for serious adverse hepatic effects associated with antipsychotics comes from controlled trials and spontaneous adverse reaction reports. However, due to the rarity of these reactions and the limits inherent in controlled trials and spontaneous reporting of serious adverse events, it is generally not possible to accurately estimate or compare the risk of serious adverse hepatic effects among different antipsychotics.

Second-generation antipsychotic agents

Aripiprazole

In premarketing clinical trials, the rate of hepatic enzyme elevation was found to be between 0.1% and 1.0%. Hepatitis and jaundice were reported as rare (<0.1%). No published case reports of hepatotoxicity are known [8].

Clozapine

Asymptomatic elevated liver enzymes have been reported in 30–50% of patients receiving clozapine, whereas serious adverse events are rare (icteric hepatitis: 84 cases out of 136 000; fatal acute fulminant hepatitis 0.001%) [9].

Table 1.7.1 Normal values of liver function tests [7]

Liver function test	Normal values	Comment
Alkaline phosphatase (ALP)[a]	30–120 U/l[b]	Elevated by cholestasis and other hepatic and non-hepatic organ damage
Aspartate aminotransferase (AST)[a]	0–35 U/l[b]	Sensitive indicator of hepatocellular damage; also found in other tissues (e.g. heart, skeletal muscle, lungs, kidneys, brain)
Alanine aminotransferase (ALT)[a]	0–35 U/l[b]	Found primarily in the liver; a sensitive indicator of hepatocellular damage
Gamma-glutamyl transpeptidase (GGT)[a]	1–94 U/l[b]	Elevated by cholestasis and acute alcohol ingestion
Albumin	35–55 g/l	Decreased with chronic hepatic problems
International normalized ratio (INR)	1–2	Elevation is suggestive of severe hepatic damage (when other causes are ruled out)
Bilirubin: Total direct Conjugated indirect Unconjugated	5.1–17 μmol/l 1.7–5.1 μmol/l 3.4–12.0 μmol/l	Conjugated and unconjugated fractions are typically elevated in cholestatic and hepatocellular liver damage

[a] ALP, ALT, AST, and GGT are the main enzymes of concern with antipsychotics; screening for adverse hepatic effects can be restricted to these tests. Further investigation may be warranted if evidence of hepatic damage is found.
[b] Varies with assay.

In a prospective inpatient study, the hepatic safety of clozapine and haloperidol were assessed weekly for the first 18 weeks of treatment, followed by monthly monitoring. The rate of hepatic enzyme elevation (alkaline phosphatase [ALP], alanine transaminase [ALT], aspartate aminotransferase [AST], gamma-glutamyl transpeptidase [GGT]) of greater than or equal to twice the ULN was higher with clozapine (37%) compared with haloperidol (17%). Most elevations were observed within the first 6 weeks of treatment; over 60% returned to normal within 13 weeks of continued treatment [10].

A fatal case of fulminant hepatic failure associated with clozapine was recently reported in an adult woman with paranoid schizophrenia and catatonic features. Hepatic enzymes were extremely elevated 6 weeks into treatment with clozapine (300 mg/day), which was discontinued immediately. Not a candidate for transplantation, she subsequently developed multiple complications leading to respiratory distress, multiorgan failure, and death 3 months after starting clozapine [11].

Olanzapine

In premarketing clinical trials ($n = 2280$), the incidences of elevated aminotransferases above 120 IU/l, 200 IU/l, and 400 IU/l were 5.9%, 1.9%, and 0.2%, respectively. None experienced elevations of AST >700 U/l, nor did any demonstrate clinical signs of hepatic impairment. Most increases were observed within 6 weeks, and no patient demonstrated clinical signs of hepatic impairment. Of 134 patients with elevations greater than twice baseline, 20 discontinued treatment [12].

In a 28-week randomized controlled trial of olanzapine versus risperidone ($n = 339$), significantly more patients experienced increases in liver transaminases with olanzapine ($p = 0.019$). None experienced clinical symptoms of hepatic disease [13].

Olanzapine was associated with a hypersensitivity reaction, consisting of fever, rash, pruritus, and hepatotoxicity (lactate dehydrogenase [LDH] 1285 IU/l, GGT 800 IU/l, AST 80 IU/l, and ALP 160 IU/l) in a 34-year-old man. Liver biopsy findings were consistent with toxic hepatitis. Hepatic function tests returned to normal 3 months after discontinuing olanzapine and starting risperidone [14].

In another report, a 78-year-old woman developed acute hepatocellular-cholestatic liver injury 13 days after starting olanzapine 10 mg/day. She presented with fever, malaise, arthralgia, upper abdominal pain, anorexia, nausea, and elevated liver function tests (AST 361–964 IU/l, ALT 204–965 IU/l, ALP 189–488 IU/l, and total bilirubin 22–156 µmol/l). Within 1 month of stopping olanzapine, she was asymptomatic and liver function tests were normal [15].

There is also a report of a case of symptomatic hepatic injury with delayed onset. After 3 years of treatment with olanzapine (10 mg/day), a 44-year-old woman presented with loss of appetite, upper abdominal pain, nausea, malaise, and hepatic enzyme elevation (AST 471 IU/l, ALT 710 IU/l, GGT 56 IU/l). Resolution occurred over 3 weeks after treatment discontinuation [16].

Paliperidone

Paliperidone is the active metabolite of risperidone and is primarily renally eliminated. For potential adverse hepatic effects, refer to the summary and monitoring recommendations for risperidone.

Quetiapine

Based on 1892 patients with baseline AST <60 IU/l included in premarketing clinical trials, the incidences of elevated aminotransferases above 120 IU/l, 200 IU/l, and 400 IU/l were 5.3%, 1.5%, and 0.2%, respectively. None experienced clinical signs of hepatic impairment. Most increases were observed within 2 months. In 80% of cases, enzymes returned to normal without intervention. Of 101 patients with elevations greater than twice the baseline value, 40 patients discontinued treatment [17].

A 58-year-old woman treated with quetiapine developed hepatic failure within 1 month of starting treatment and died 3 weeks after being hospitalized.

Routine monitoring and physical examination revealed severely elevated liver enzymes, mild hepatomegaly and splenomegaly, edema of the lower extremities, and mild asterixis. The patient's condition further deteriorated with encephalopathy, hepatocyte necrosis, sepsis, renal failure, coma, and death [18].

Reversible cholestasis was observed in a 30-year-old man within 3 weeks of exposure to quetiapine. He originally developed reversible cholestasis after 8 years of risperidone therapy. Preceding trials of olanzapine and ziprasidone were uneventful [19].

In another case, hepatitis was reported in a 21-year-old male initiated on quetiapine 300 mg/day for only 3 days before symptom onset. He presented with fatigue, nausea, vomiting, abdominal pain, and palpitations for 1 week. Laboratory tests revealed total bilirubin 14.7 mg/dl, direct bilirubin 7.3 mg/dl, ALT 2582 IU/l, AST 1659 IU/l, and ALP 167 IU/l. Liver biopsy was compatible with drug-induced hepatitis [20].

Risperidone

Risperidone has been associated with several pediatric cases of hepatotoxicity. Presentation has been similar to non-alcoholic steatohepatitis. In some cases, liver enzymes returned to normal upon discontinuation of risperidone and concomitant weight loss [21,22].

Acute-onset risperidone-induced cholestatic hepatitis has been reported in three adults. Liver enzymes increased within 5–30 days of risperidone initiation. In one case, liver biopsy performed 48 days after starting risperidone was consistent with drug-induced cholestatic hepatitis. In the second case, liver enzymes normalized within 30 days of risperidone discontinuation, although weight gain of 20 kg may have been a confounding factor. In the third case, a 64-year-old man also treated with fluoxetine had an increase in liver enzymes after only four doses of risperidone 2 mg/day. Liver enzymes normalized within 2 weeks of a switch from risperidone to haloperidol [23–25].

Risperidone has also been associated with a late-onset case of cholestasis, after eight years of treatment. Signs and symptoms resolved with the discontinuation of risperidone [19].

A case of risperidone-induced hepatitis and pancreatitis was reported in a 32-year-old woman. Within 1 week of initiating risperidone, symptoms of nausea, vomiting, abdominal pain, and anorexia, in conjunction with jaundice, dark urine, and elevations of AST, ALT, GGT, ALP, total bilirubin, and amylase were noted. Laboratory measures improved significantly within 1 week of stopping risperidone [26].

Among three cases of risperidone-associated hepatotoxicity in the elderly, the onset of signs and symptoms varied markedly (2 days, 6 weeks, and 7 months). In each case, hepatic functioning normalized shortly after discontinuation of risperidone [27,28].

Ziprasidone

No reports of hepatic injury with ziprasidone have been identified other than in the product monograph, which indicates that hepatitis, hepatomegaly, and fatty liver deposits are rare adverse events [29].

First-generation antipsychotic agents

Chlorpromazine

The incidence of chlorpromazine-associated elevations of ALT is 25–50% and the rate of clinically significant cholestatic hepatotoxicity is estimated to be 0.1–1%. Symptoms typically appear within 1–5 weeks. Laboratory findings include increased bilirubin, ALP, and transaminases [30].

Other phenothiazines

A case–control comparison found increased risk of hepatotoxicity with aliphatic (e.g. chlorpromazine), piperidine (e.g. thioridazine), and piperazine (e.g. trifluoperazine) phenothiazine derivatives. The rate of clinically significant hepatotoxicity is estimated to be 0.5–2% [31].

Haloperidol

While transient transaminase elevation may be common with haloperidol (~15%), hepatotoxicity is rare, affecting approximately 0.002% of haloperidol-treated patients. The average onset of hepatotoxicity is 4–5 weeks from initiation of treatment [30,32,33].

Monitoring

It is recommended that hepatic functioning be assessed at baseline and 1 month after starting an antipsychotic. Testing should include hepatocellular and biliary functioning (e.g. ALP, ALT, AST, and GGT). Follow-up and/or expanded monitoring is required if abnormalities are found.

Other routine monitoring of hepatic function is not recommended with antipsychotic treatment in the absence of clinical suspicion. If the patient has other risk factors for hepatic problems (e.g. alcohol or substance abuse, viral hepatitis), these should guide monitoring of hepatic function.

Symptoms meriting investigation in individuals with abnormal liver function tests include itching, dark urine, pale stools, abnormal bruising or bleeding, confusion, nausea, vomiting or diarrhea, fever with chills, malaise, fatigue, muscle aches, and abdominal pain.

Signs of liver disease include icterus, hepatomegaly, hepatic tenderness, splenomegaly, spider angiomata, palmar erythema, and excoriations.

When antipsychotic-induced hepatic damage is suspected based on laboratory and clinical findings, other laboratory measures including bilirubin tests and determination of the international normalized ratio (INR) may be warranted.

REFERENCES

1. Farkas J, Farkas P, Hyde D. Liver and gastroenterology tests. In Lee M, American Society of Health-System Pharmacists, ed., *Basic Skills in Interpreting Laboratory Data*, 3rd edn. Bethesda, MD: American Society of Health-System Pharmacists; 2004.
2. Diehl AM. Hepatic complications of obesity. *Gastroenterol Clin North Am* 2005;**34**(1):45–61.
3. Arana GW. An overview of side effects caused by typical antipsychotics. *J Clin Psychiatry* 2000;**61** Suppl. 8:5–11; discussion 12–3.

Monitoring schedule for **ANTIPSYCHOTIC-INDUCED HEPATIC EFFECTS**

Monitoring includes assessment of baseline, new-onset, or changes in liver enzymes and liver function tests. AST, ALT, ALP, and GGT are the main enzymes of concern; screening can be restricted to these tests.

	Baseline	Weeks		Months					Long-term monitoring
		1	2	1	2	3	6	12	
Second-generation antipsychotics									
Aripiprazole	•			•					(★)
Clozapine	•			•					(★)
Olanzapine	•			•					(★)
Paliperidone	•			•					(★)
Quetiapine	•			•					(★)
Risperidone	•			•					(★)
Ziprasidone	•			•					(★)
First-generation antipsychotics									
Chlorpromazine	•			•					(★)
Flupenthixol	•			•					(★)
Fluphenazine	•			•					(★)
Haloperidol	•			•					(★)
Loxapine	•			•					(★)
Methotrimeprazine	•			•					(★)
Molindone	•			•					(★)
Pericyazine	•			•					(★)
Perphenazine	•			•					(★)
Pimozide	•			•					(★)
Pipotiazine palmitate	•			•					(★)
Thioridazine	•			•					(★)
Thiothixene	•			•					(★)
Trifluoperazine	•			•					(★)
Zuclopenthixol	•			•					(★)

• Monitor for adverse effect. (★) As clinically indicated.

4. Bénichou C. *Adverse Drug Reactions : a Practical Guide to Diagnosis and Management*. New York, NY: J. Wiley & Sons; 1994.

5. Oyewumi LK, De Wit R. *Managing Side Effects of Psychotropic Drugs: a Clinical Handbook for Health Care Professionals*. London, ON: Zxmaxx Communications; 1998.

6. Cuffel BJ, Heithoff KA, Lawson W. Correlates of patterns of substance abuse among patients with schizophrenia. *Hosp Community Psychiatry* 1993;**44**(3):247–51.

7. Kratz A, Ferraro M, Sluss PM, Lewandrowski KB. Case records of the Massachusetts General Hospital. Weekly clinicopathological exercises. Laboratory reference values. *N Engl J Med* 2004;**351**(15):1548–63.

8. Bristol-Myers Squibb, Otsuka America Pharmaceutical. *Abilify (Aripiprazole) U.S. Full Prescribing Information*. Tokyo, Japan: Otsuka Pharmaceutical Co., Ltd.; 2008.

9. Macfarlane B, Davies S, Mannan K, Sarsam R, Pariente D, Dooley J. Fatal acute fulminant liver failure due to clozapine: a case report and review of clozapine-induced hepatotoxicity. *Gastroenterology* 1997;**112**(5):1707–9.

10. Hummer M, Kurz M, Kurzthaler I, Oberbauer H, Miller C, Fleischhacker WW. Hepatotoxicity of clozapine. *J Clin Psychopharmacol* 1997;**17**(4):314–17.

11. Chang A, Krygier DS, Chatur N, Yoshida EM. Clozapine-induced fatal fulminant hepatic failure: a case report. *Can J Gastroenterol* 2009;**23**(5):376–8.

12. Canadian Pharmacists Association. Zyprexa (olanzapine) product monograph. In Canadian Pharmacists Association, ed., *Compendium of Pharmaceuticals and Specialties*. Toronto; 2006.

13. Tran PV, Hamilton SH, Kuntz AJ, et al. Double-blind comparison of olanzapine versus risperidone in the treatment of schizophrenia and other psychotic disorders. *J Clin Psychopharmacol* 1997;**17**(5):407–18.

14. Raz A, Bergman R, Eilam O, Yungerman T, Hayek T. A case report of olanzapine-induced hypersensitivity syndrome. *Am J Med Sci* 2001;**321**(2):156–8.

15. Jadallah KA, Limauro DL, Colatrella AM. Acute hepatocellular-cholestatic liver injury after olanzapine therapy. *Ann Intern Med* 2003;**138**(4):357–8.

16. Ozcanli T, Erdogan A, Ozdemir S, et al. Severe liver enzyme elevations after three years of olanzapine treatment: a case report and review of olanzapine associated hepatotoxicity. *Prog Neuropsychopharmacol Biol Psychiatry* 2006;**30**(6):1163–6.

17. Canadian Pharmacists Association. Seroquel (quetiapine) product monograph. In Canadian Pharmacists Association, ed., *Compendium of Pharmaceuticals and Specialties*. Toronto; 2006.

18. El Hajj I, Sharara AI, Rockey DC. Subfulminant liver failure associated with quetiapine. *Eur J Gastroenterol Hepatol* 2004;**16**(12):1415–18.

19. Wright TM, Vandenberg AM. Risperidone- and quetiapine-induced cholestasis. *Ann Pharmacother* 2007;**41**(9):1518–23.

20. Shpaner A, Li W, Ankoma-Sey V, Botero RC. Drug-induced liver injury: hepatotoxicity of quetiapine revisited. *Eur J Gastroenterol Hepatol* 2008;**20**(11):1106–9.

21. Landau J, Martin A. Is liver function monitoring warranted during risperidone treatment? *J Am Acad Child Adolesc Psychiatry* 1998;**37**(10):1007–8.

22. Kumra S, Herion D, Jacobsen LK, Briguglia C, Grothe D. Case study: risperidone-induced hepatotoxicity in pediatric patients. *J Am Acad Child Adolesc Psychiatry* 1997;**36**(5):701–5.

23. Benazzi F. Risperidone-induced hepatotoxicity. *Pharmacopsychiatry* 1998;**31**(6):241.

24. Krebs S, Dormann H, Muth-Selbach U, Hahn EG, Brune K, Schneider HT. Risperidone-induced cholestatic hepatitis. *Eur J Gastroenterol Hepatol* 2001;**13**(1):67–9.

25. Llinares Tello F, Hernandez Prats C, Bosacoma Ros N, et al. Acute cholestatic hepatitis probably associated with risperidone. *Int J Psychiatry Med* 2005;**35**(2):199–205.

26. Cordeiro Q, Jr, Elkis H. Pancreatitis and cholestatic hepatitis induced by risperidone. *J Clin Psychopharmacol* 2001;**21**(5):529–30.

27. Fuller MA, Simon MR, Freedman L. Risperidone-associated hepatotoxicity. *J Clin Psychopharmacol* 1996;**16**(1):84–5.

28. Phillips EJ, Liu BA, Knowles SR. Rapid onset of risperidone-induced hepatotoxicity. *Ann Pharmacother* 1998;**32**(7–8):843.

29. Pfizer Canada Inc. *Zeldox (Ziprasidone hydrochloride) Canadian Product Monograph*. Quebec, Canada: Pfizer Canada Inc.; 2007.

30. Selim K, Kaplowitz N. Hepatotoxicity of psychotropic drugs. *Hepatology* 1999 May;**29**(5):1347–51.

31. Jones JK, Van de Carr SW, Zimmerman H, Leroy A. Hepatotoxicity associated with phenothiazines. *Psychopharmacol Bull* 1983;**19**(1):24–7.

32. Dincsoy HP, Saelinger DA. Haloperidol-induced chronic cholestatic liver disease. *Gastroenterology* 1982;**83**(3):694–700.

33. Dumortier G, Cabaret W, Stamatiadis L, et al. Hepatic tolerance of atypical antipsychotic drugs. *Encephale* 2002;**28**(6):542–51.

Neuroleptic malignant syndrome

Background

Neuroleptic malignant syndrome (NMS) is an uncommon, severe, and potentially life-threatening adverse effect of antipsychotics. Previous rates reported from prospective studies ranged from 0.07% to 1.1%; however, more recent data suggest a lower incidence of 0.01–0.02%. The case fatality rate is estimated at 10% [1–3].

Several risk factors, including exhaustion, agitation, dehydration, restraint, low iron, and in particular a history of NMS, have been proposed, but few are well established. Although NMS is rare with all antipsychotics, the risk appears highest with high-potency first-generation antipsychotics and lowest with newer, low-potency second-generation agents. A higher daily dose and rate of titration may also increase risk [1,2,4].

The pathoetiology of NMS appears to relate to a relative dopamine hypofunctionality as the majority of cases are caused by dopamine antagonists (e.g. antipsychotics). Of note, a similar syndrome can result from the abrupt discontinuation of dopaminergic agents [2].

Neuroleptic malignant syndrome is characterized by severe rigidity, tremor, fever, altered mental status, and autonomic dysfunction. Common laboratory changes include an elevated white blood cell count and a sometimes markedly elevated creatine kinase (CK). Variant forms may exist in which one or more classic features, for example hyperthermia or marked rigidity, are absent. Other laboratory findings can include elevations in transaminases and lactate dehydrogenase, metabolic acidosis, hypoxia, and reduced iron concentration [1,2,5,6].

Neuroleptic malignant syndrome is a diagnosis of exclusion with an extensive differential diagnosis covering infectious, endocrine, environmental, psychiatric, neurological, and other toxicological etiologies. The onset of signs and symptoms may be useful in making the diagnosis. Alterations in mental status and other neurological signs generally precede the onset of more systemic signs. Onset is generally gradual (although not always), worsening over two or more days [2].

Nearly all cases of NMS develop within the first few days to weeks of the start of antipsychotic treatment, although some may have a later onset with a change in dose or agent [7].

Neuroleptic malignant syndrome is considered to be a potentially fatal psychiatric emergency requiring an inpatient hospital stay, often in intensive care. Antipsychotic treatment should be stopped immediately. For most people, the syndrome is self-limiting with recovery typically taking 1–2 weeks [7].

Virtually all antipsychotic drugs have been associated with NMS, presumably caused by dopamine receptor antagonism. However, the incidence appears to be dropping with the increased use of second-generation agents. A variant form of NMS, with less severe extrapyramidal symptoms (EPS), has been reported with selected second-generation agents [2,8,9].

Agents of interest

All antipsychotics are considered to be liable to cause NMS. Non-antipsychotic dopamine D_2 receptor antagonists (such as metoclopramide) have also been associated with NMS [1].

Monitoring schedule for **NEUROLEPTIC MALIGNANT SYNDROME**

At baseline, assess for the presence of abnormal tone and other clinical features of EPS and NMS. Determine if there is a history of NMS. Regular monitoring includes assessment of signs and symptoms consistent with NMS (severe rigidity, tremor, fever, altered mental status, autonomic dysfunction, elevated CK, and elevated white blood cells).

| | Baseline | Weeks | | Months | | | | | | Long-term monitoring |
		1	2	1	2	3	6	12	
Second-generation antipsychotics										
Aripiprazole	•									(★)
Clozapine	•									(★)
Olanzapine	•									(★)
Paliperidone	•									(★)
Quetiapine	•									(★)
Risperidone	•									(★)
Ziprasidone	•									(★)
First-generation antipsychotics										
Chlorpromazine	•									(★)
Flupenthixol	•									(★)
Fluphenazine	•									(★)
Haloperidol	•									(★)
Loxapine	•									(★)
Methotrimeprazine	•									(★)
Molindone	•									(★)
Pericyazine	•									(★)
Perphenazine	•									(★)
Pimozide	•									(★)
Pipotiazine palmitate	•									(★)
Thioridazine	•									(★)
Thiothixene	•									(★)
Trifluoperazine	•									(★)
Zuclopenthixol	•									(★)

• Monitor for adverse effect. (★) As clinically indicated.

A second-generation form of NMS, consisting of less severe EPS and less extreme elevations in CK, has been proposed and was thought to occur more often with second-generation antipsychotics. Presently, there is insufficient evidence to establish this as a variant form of NMS [5,10,11].

Monitoring

It is difficult to estimate antipsychotic-specific risks due to the infrequency of NMS. Therefore, monitoring recommendations apply equally to all agents. It should be noted that EPS may be a less prominent manifestation of NMS in patients taking low-potency second-generation agents (e.g. clozapine, quetiapine).

Before initiating any antipsychotic agent, it is important to assess the patient for a history of NMS and for the presence of abnormal muscle tone at baseline.

Collaborative efforts are needed to ensure that early indicators of NMS are identified. This requires the appropriate education of caregivers about the early warning signs of NMS.

Summary of what to monitor

As clinically indicated, NMS should be suspected if the following signs and symptoms are present:
- Fever
- Muscle rigidity unresponsive to anticholinergics, ranging from hypertonicity to severe lead pipe rigidity
- Other movement problems (tremor, abnormal reflexes, bradykinesia, chorea, dystonias)
- Altered level of consciousness (ranges from a decreased awareness of one's surroundings to obtundation)
- Agitation
- Autonomic dysfunction (hypertension, postural hypotension, labile blood pressure, tachycardia, tachypnea, diaphoresis, sialorrhea, skin pallor, urinary incontinence)
- Creatine kinase levels above 5000 IU are common
- Leukocyte count is frequently elevated

REFERENCES

1. Pelonero AL, Levenson JL, Pandurangi AK. Neuroleptic malignant syndrome. In Young RR, Joseph AB, eds., *Movement Disorders in Neurology and Neuropsychiatry*, 3rd edn. Malden, MA: Blackwell Science, Inc.; 1999.
2. Strawn JR, Keck PE, Jr, Caroff SN. Neuroleptic malignant syndrome. *Am J Psychiatry* 2007;**164**(6):870–6.
3. Stubner S, Rustenbeck E, Grohmann R, et al. Severe and uncommon involuntary movement disorders due to psychotropic drugs. *Pharmacopsychiatry* 2004;**37** Suppl. 1: S54–64.
4. Rosebush PI, Mazurek MF. Serum iron and neuroleptic malignant syndrome. *Lancet* 1991;**338**(8760):149–51.
5. Hasan S, Buckley P. Novel antipsychotics and the neuroleptic malignant syndrome: a review and critique. *Am J Psychiatry* 1998;**155**(8):1113–6.
6. Picard LS, Lindsay S, Strawn JR, Kaneria RM, Patel NC, Keck PE, Jr. Atypical neuroleptic malignant syndrome: Diagnostic controversies and considerations. *Pharmacotherapy* 2008;**28**(4):530–5.
7. Caroff SN. Neuroleptic malignant syndrome: still a risk, but which patients may be in danger? *Curr Psychiatry* 2003;**2**:36–42.
8. Tarsy D, Baldessarini RJ. Epidemiology of tardive dyskinesia: is risk declining with modern antipsychotics? *Mov Disord* 2006;**21**(5):589–98.
9. Karaganis J, Phillips L, Hogan K, LeDrew K. Re: neuroleptic malignant syndrome associated with quetiapine. *Can J Psychiatry* 2001;**46**(4):370–1.
10. Sachdev P, Kruk J, Kneebone M, Kissane D. Clozapine-induced neuroleptic malignant syndrome: review and report of new cases. *J Clin Psychopharmacol* 1995;**15**(5):365–71.
11. Ananth J, Parameswaran S, Gunatilake S, Burgoyne K, Sidhom T. Neuroleptic malignant syndrome and atypical antipsychotic drugs. *J Clin Psychiatry* 2004;**65**(4):464–70.

Obesity and weight gain

Background

The prevalence of being overweight or obese is higher in patients with psychotic disorders than in the general population, relating at least in part to a combination of excessive food intake, poor diet composition, and low physical activity [1].

Fat distribution differs between people with and without schizophrenia. In one comparative study, abdominal fat volume was three times higher in treatment-naive patients with schizophrenia ($n = 19$) compared with age- and gender-matched healthy controls ($n = 19$), despite similar baseline body mass indexes (BMIs) (24.6 vs. 23.0) [2].

Weight fluctuates during the course of schizophrenia. During times of worsening disease, weight and appetite tend to decrease. Conversely, as acute psychotic episodes subside, it has been noted that weight and appetite tend to either increase or return to baseline [3,4].

Several but not all newer antipsychotic agents have been associated with sometimes marked weight gain [3,5–9].

The mechanism by which antipsychotic agents cause weight gain is unclear, but several hypotheses have been proposed. One of the strongest associations with weight gain is the antipsychotic's binding affinity for H_1 receptors (see Table 1.21.1 on p.142), which is associated with a change in eating behaviors and a decreased sensation of satiety [9].

Genetic studies suggest that an interaction between genetic susceptibility and antipsychotic pharmacology predict weight gain. Findings have implicated genes linked to serotonergic ($5\text{-}HT_{2c}$) and adrenergic (α_{2a})

mechanisms as well as leptin, guanine nucleotide binding protein (GNB3), synaptomal-associated protein 25 kDa (SNAP25), and several other targets [10–13].

Antipsychotics have different binding affinities to several receptors associated with weight gain, and details on their effects on gene expression are helping to explain the observed variances in weight gain liability. For example, aripiprazole's low weight gain potential may relate to its lack of antagonism at serotonin $5\text{-}HT_{2c}$ receptors and moderate affinity at histamine H_1 receptors, whereas olanzapine and clozapine are potent antagonists at both of these receptors [13].

Body mass index is weight in kilograms divided by height in meters squared (kg/m^2). It is an indicator of total body fat and is valid in both men and women. Body fat may be overestimated in those with a muscular build (e.g. athletes), and may be underestimated in those with low muscle mass (e.g. elderly patients). Body mass index is classified as underweight, normal, overweight, and obese (see Tables 1.9.1 and 1.9.2) [14,15].

The clinical ramifications of weight gain are many. Weight gain, especially to the point of obesity, has been associated with hypertension, hyperlipidemia, type 2 diabetes, coronary heart disease, stroke, osteoarthritis, sleep apnea, gallbladder disease, some cancers (colorectal and prostate in men, and breast, cervical, endometrial, gall bladder, and ovarian in women), and several other conditions [16,17].

Waist size is a useful and simple indicator of risk. Men and women with a waist circumference (WC) of greater than 40 in (102 cm) and 35 in (88 cm), respectively, are at increased risk for hypertension, type 2 diabetes, dyslipidemia, and metabolic syndrome [14,15,18].

Table 1.9.1 Weight categories and disease risk by BMI and waist circumference [15]

Category	BMI (kg/m^2)	Men, WC ≤40 in (102 cm)^b Women, WC ≤35 in (88 cm)	Men, WC ≥40 in (102 cm)^b Women, WC ≥35 in (88 cm)
		Disease risk^a (relative to normal weight and waist circumference [WC])	
Underweight	<18.5		
Normal^c	18.5–24.9		
Overweight	25.0–29.9	Increased	High
Obese:			
Mild	30.0–34.9	High	Very high
Moderate	35.0–39.9	Very high	Very high
Severe or extreme	≥40.0	Extremely high	Extremely high

^{a} For type 2 diabetes, hypertension, and cardiovascular disease.
^{b} Waist circumference cut-off points may be lower in some populations (e.g. older individuals, Asian population), especially in the presence of features of metabolic syndrome (e.g. hypertriglyceridemia).
^{c} Increased waist circumference can be a marker for increased risk even in individuals of normal weight.

Besides having an impact on physical health, antipsychotic-induced weight gain can negatively affect psychological health (e.g. self-esteem, self-worth), and in turn may lead to reduced adherence or treatment rejection. This can result in an increased risk of relapse and longer hospital stays [3,15–17,19].

Risk factors for antipsychotic-induced weight gain

Weight gain is most rapid in the early weeks of therapy. For some agents, weight gain can plateau after the first few months of therapy (e.g. risperidone, quetiapine, and ziprasidone), while for other agents it may continue well beyond 20 weeks (e.g. olanzapine and clozapine) [20].

Evidence is inconclusive as to whether links exist between antipsychotic-associated weight gain and antipsychotic dose, clinical response, age, sex, or baseline BMI. To date, there are no reliable predictors of antipsychotic-induced weight gain [19].

Agents of interest

Differences in research methodologies, (e.g. different patient populations, length of studies, dosages used,

etc.) and significant inter-patient variation make it difficult to ascertain the true impact that antipsychotic agents have on weight.

Second-generation antipsychotic agents

Aripiprazole

Acute and long-term treatment trials indicate that aripiprazole is associated with little or no weight gain [9,21].

Switching trials show weight loss when patients are switched from olanzapine to aripiprazole [9,22,23].

The manufacturer reports that clinically significant weight gain (≥7% increase in baseline weight) has been observed at a rate of 8% [24].

Clozapine

Evidence linking clozapine to weight gain is significant [5,25].

Patients using clozapine can average 8.8–11 lb (4–5 kg) of weight gain over 10 weeks [5].

Clozapine-induced weight gain can continue for 4 years before it plateaus. Most of the weight gain occurs within the first year of medication use [25].

Olanzapine

Evidence linking olanzapine to weight gain is significant [5].

Olanzapine-associated weight gain is comparable to that associated with clozapine [5,7].

In the CATIE trial (a large, double-blind, 18-month, randomized trial that compared olanzapine, risperidone, quetiapine, perphenazine, and ziprasidone therapy in patients who were previously on a variety of antipsychotics), olanzapine was associated with the highest rate (30%) of clinically significant weight gain (≥7% increase in baseline weight). Quetiapine was second at a rate of 16%. The average rate of weight increase with olanzapine was 2.0 lb (0.9 kg) per month (range: –1.4 to 9.5 lb [–0.6 to 4.3 kg] per month). The second highest rate was 0.5 lb (0.2 kg) per month observed with quetiapine [8].

An earlier meta-analysis estimated an 8.8 lb (4 kg) mean weight increase with olanzapine over 10 weeks [5].

It has been estimated that approximately 45% of patients on olanzapine will develop clinically important weight gain (i.e. ≥7% total body weight) over 1.5 years of treatment, a rate that is 2.5 times greater than the rate associated with haloperidol use [26].

The results of the CAFE trial (a double-blind randomized trial of first-episode psychosis patients [$n = 400$]) confirmed concerns of clinically significant weight gain with newer antipsychotics, especially olanzapine. Rates of ≥7% increase in baseline weight at 12 and 24 weeks were: olanzapine 60% and 80%; quetiapine 29% and 50%; and risperidone 32% and 58% [27].

Paliperidone

The manufacturer reports that clinically significant weight gain (≥7% increase in baseline weight) was observed in brief (6-week), placebo-controlled, fixed-dose studies at rates of 6–9% among doses ranging from 3 mg/day to 12 mg/day [28].

Weight gain with paliperidone is not expected to be greater than with risperidone and may be similar.

Quetiapine

In the CATIE trial, 16% of participants taking quetiapine experienced clinically significant weight gain (≥7%

increase in baseline weight). The rate of weight change was 0.5 lb (0.2 kg) per month (range: –4.4 to 6.3 lb [–2 to 2.9 kg] per month) [8].

In the CAFE trial, weight gain at 1 year of follow-up with quetiapine (12.5 lb [5.7 kg]) was similar to risperidone (14.5 lb [6.6 kg]) and significantly less than with olanzapine (24.4 lb [11.1 kg]). The rate of clinically significant weight gain (≥7%) with quetiapine was 50% compared with 58% with risperidone and 80% with olanzapine [27].

Risperidone

Evidence linking risperidone to weight gain is significant [5].

The CATIE trial reported that 14% of patients treated with risperidone experienced a weight increase of ≥7% from baseline. The median change in weight was 0.0 lb (range: –24 to +24 lb [–11 to + 11 kg]) [8].

Weight gain at 10 weeks of treatment is estimated to be approximately 4.4 lb (2 kg) [5].

Approximately 30% of patients on risperidone will develop significant weight gain (i.e. ≥7% total body weight) within 2 years – a rate 1.5 times greater than the rate associated with haloperidol use [26].

In first-episode psychosis patients, the CAFE trial found that weight gain was similar between risperidone and quetiapine and significantly greater with olanzapine. Weight gains at 12 and 24 weeks, respectively, were: olanzapine 16 lb (7.1 kg) and 24 lb (11.1 kg); quetiapine 8 lb (3.7 kg) and 12 lb (5.7 kg); and risperidone 9 lb (4 kg) and 14 (6.6 kg) [27].

Ziprasidone

In the CATIE trial, 7% of ziprasidone-treated patients had a significant weight gain (≥7% increase from baseline). The median change in weight was –2 lb (–0.9 kg) (range –24 to +18 lb [–11 to +8.2 kg]). Overall weight loss may reflect switches from antipsychotics with high weight gain liability [8].

At 10 weeks of treatment, no change in weight is expected with ziprasidone [5].

Monitoring schedule for **ANTIPSYCHOTIC-INDUCED WEIGHT GAIN AND OBESITY**

Monitoring should include documentation and tracking of weight, waist circumference, and body mass index.

	Baseline	Weeks		Months					Long-term monitoring
		1	2	1	2	3	6	12	
Second-generation antipsychotics									
Aripiprazole	•			•		•	•	•	★ ⑥
Clozapine	•		•	•	•	•	•	•	★ ③
Olanzapine	•		•	•	•	•	•	•	★ ③
Paliperidone	•		•	•	•	•	•	•	★ ③
Quetiapine	•		•	•	•	•	•	•	★ ③
Risperidone	•		•	•	•	•	•	•	★ ③
Ziprasidone	•			•		•	•	•	★ ⑥
First-generation antipsychotics									
Chlorpromazine	•		•	•	•	•		•	★ ③
Flupenthixol	•			•		•			★ ⑥
Fluphenazine	•			•		•			★ ⑥
Haloperidol	•			•		•			★ ⑥
Loxapine	•			•		•			★ ⑥
Methotrimeprazine	•		•	•	•	•	•	•	★ ③
Molindone	•			•		•			★ ⑥
Pericyazine	•			•		•			★ ⑥
Perphenazine	•		•	•	•	•	•	•	★ ③
Pimozide	•			•		•			★ ⑥
Pipotiazine palmitate	•			•		•			★ ⑥
Thioridazine	•		•	•	•	•	•	•	★ ③
Thiothixene	•			•		•			★ ⑥
Trifluoperazine	•			•		•			★ ⑥
Zuclopenthixol	•			•		•			★ ⑥

• Monitor for adverse effect. ★ As clinically indicated. ③ Every 3 months. ⑥ Every 6 months.

Table 1.9.2 BMI chart[a]

BMI	19	20	21	22	23	24	25	26	27	28	29	30	31	32	33	34	35
Height (in)								Body weight (lb)									
58	91	96	100	105	110	115	119	124	129	134	138	143	148	153	158	162	167
59	94	99	104	109	114	119	124	128	133	138	143	148	153	158	163	168	173
60	97	102	107	112	118	123	128	133	138	143	148	153	158	163	168	174	179
61	100	106	111	116	122	127	132	137	143	148	153	158	164	169	174	180	185
62	104	109	115	120	126	131	136	142	147	153	158	164	169	175	180	186	191
63	107	113	118	124	130	135	141	146	152	158	163	169	175	180	186	191	197
64	110	116	122	128	134	140	145	151	157	163	169	174	180	186	192	197	204
65	114	120	126	132	138	144	150	156	162	168	174	180	186	192	198	204	210
66	118	124	130	136	142	148	155	161	167	173	179	186	192	198	204	210	216
67	121	127	134	140	146	153	159	166	172	178	185	191	198	204	211	217	223
68	125	131	138	144	151	158	164	171	177	184	190	197	203	210	216	223	230
69	128	135	142	149	155	162	169	176	182	189	196	203	209	216	223	230	236
70	132	139	146	153	160	167	174	181	188	195	202	209	216	222	229	236	243
71	136	143	150	157	165	172	179	186	193	200	208	215	222	229	236	243	250
72	140	147	154	162	169	177	184	191	199	206	213	221	228	235	242	250	258
73	144	151	159	166	174	182	189	197	204	212	219	227	235	242	250	257	265
74	148	155	163	171	179	186	194	202	210	218	225	233	241	249	256	264	272
75	152	160	168	176	184	192	200	208	216	224	232	240	248	256	264	272	279
76	156	164	172	180	189	197	205	213	221	230	238	246	254	263	271	279	287

Note: 1 lb = 0.454 kg; 1 in = 0.0254 m.

[a] Does not apply to children and teenagers, as their body fat changes with growth; for these populations, an age- and sex-based BMI (i.e. BMI-for-age) best represents their BMI category. For calculations, refer to http://apps.nccd.cdc.gov/dnpabmi/.

First-generation antipsychotic agents

Chlorpromazine

Evidence linking chlorpromazine to weight gain is extensive [5].

Patients using chlorpromazine average about 4.4 lb (2 kg) of weight gain over 10 weeks [5].

Haloperidol

Evidence assessing the effect of haloperidol on weight is extensive [5,26].

Patients using haloperidol average an increase of 1.1 lb (0.5 kg) over 10 weeks and typically gain about 6.6 lb (3 kg) in 4–5 years [5,26].

Approximately 20% of patients on haloperidol develop significant weight gain (i.e. ≥7% total body weight) in 1.5 years [26].

Thioridazine

Evidence linking thioridazine to weight gain is significant [5].

Patients using thioridazine average 7.7 lb (3.5 kg) over 10 weeks [5].

Others first-generation antipsychotics

Weight gain with antipsychotics has become a prominent issue in recent years coincident with the growing use of second-generation agents. Specific data are lacking regarding the weight gain liability of many first-generation antipsychotics. In general, weight gain liability is inversely correlated to potency at dopamine receptors, with chlorpromazine and thioridazine representing the higher end of the spectrum and haloperidol the lower end.

Monitoring

Considering the high prevalence of overweight and obesity in patients who take antipsychotics long term, frequent regular monitoring of weight is recommended, regardless of antipsychotic treatment.

Monitoring weight is simple, time-efficient, and inexpensive. For almost all antipsychotics, it is recommended that weight be measured every 3 months or at every clinic visit, whichever is less frequent, during the first year of new treatment. Thereafter, weight should be recorded every 3–6 months minimally.

Body mass index and WC should also be determined. These are useful indicators of increasing risk and when interventions are required to address weight problems.

To measure WC, patients should be in the standing position with their feet 10–12 in (25–30 cm) apart and arms hanging naturally at their sides. The measuring device should be positioned horizontally at the level of the top of the iliac crest, which is used as a landmark to standardize measurement. The measurer should stand to the side of the patient and fit the tape snugly around the waist. The circumference should be measured with the patient's abdominal muscles relaxed at the end of a normal expiration [15].

Monitoring tools

The formulae used for calculation of BMI are:

Imperial: BMI = [weight (lb)/height $(in)^2$] × 703

Metric: BMI = weight (kg)/height $(m)^2$

Table 1.9.2 gives BMI values for imperial measurements.

Useful websites

- Body mass index overview and calculator:http://www.nhlbisupport.com/bmi/
- Body mass index for children and teens http://apps.nccd.cdc.gov/dnpabmi/

REFERENCES

1. Melkersson KI, Dahl ML, Hulting AL. Guidelines for prevention and treatment of adverse effects of antipsychotic drugs on glucose-insulin homeostasis and lipid metabolism. *Psychopharmacology (Berl)* 2004;**175**(1):1–6.
2. Ryan MC, Flanagan S, Kinsella U, Keeling F, Thakore JH. The effects of atypical antipsychotics on visceral fat distribution in first episode, drug-naive patients with schizophrenia. *Life Sci* 2004;**74**(16):1999–2008.
3. Allison DB, Casey DE. Antipsychotic-induced weight gain: a review of the literature. *J Clin Psychiatry* 2001;**62** Suppl. 7:22–31.
4. Koponen H, Saari K, Savolainen M, Isohanni M. Weight gain and glucose and lipid metabolism disturbances during antipsychotic medication: a review. *Eur Arch Psychiatry Clin Neurosci* 2002;**252**(6):294–8.
5. Allison DB, Mentore JL, Heo M, et al. Antipsychotic-induced weight gain: a comprehensive research synthesis. *Am J Psychiatry* 1999;**156**(11):1686–96.
6. Sussman N. Review of atypical antipsychotics and weight gain. *J Clin Psychiatry* 2001;**62** Suppl. 23:5–12.
7. Nasrallah H. A review of the effect of atypical antipsychotics on weight. *Psychoneuroendocrinology* 2003;**28** Suppl. 1:83–96.
8. Lieberman JA, Stroup TS, McEvoy JP, et al. Effectiveness of antipsychotic drugs in patients with chronic schizophrenia. *N Engl J Med* 2005;**353**(12):1209–23.
9. Newcomer JW. Antipsychotic medications: metabolic and cardiovascular risk. *J Clin Psychiatry* 2007;**68** Suppl. 4:8–13.
10. Muller DJ, Kennedy JL. Genetics of antipsychotic treatment emergent weight gain in schizophrenia. *Pharmacogenomics* 2006;**7**(6):863–87.
11. Chagnon YC. Susceptibility genes for the side effect of antipsychotics on body weight and obesity. *Curr Drug Targets* 2006;**7**(12):1681–95.
12. Reynolds GP, Hill MJ, Kirk SL. The 5-HT$_{2C}$ receptor and antipsychotic-induced weight gain – mechanisms and genetics. *J Psychopharmacol* 2006;**20**(4 Suppl.):15–18.
13. Rege S. Antipsychotic induced weight gain in schizophrenia: mechanisms and management. *Aust N Z J Psychiatry* 2008;**42**(5):369–81.
14. National Institutes of Health. Clinical guidelines on the identification, evaluation, and treatment of overweight and obesity in adults – the evidence report. *Obes Res* 1998;**6** Suppl. 2:51S–209S.

15. Lau DC, Douketis JD, Morrison KM, et al. 2006 Canadian clinical practice guidelines on the management and prevention of obesity in adults and children. *CMAJ* 2007;**176** (8 Suppl.):online 1–117.

16. Kurzthaler I, Fleischhacker WW. The clinical implications of weight gain in schizophrenia. *J Clin Psychiatry* 2001;**62** Suppl. 7:32–7.

17. Douketis JD, Feightner JW, Attia J, Feldman WF. Periodic health examination, 1999 update: 1. Detection, prevention and treatment of obesity. Canadian Task Force on Preventive Health Care. *CMAJ* 1999;**160** (4):513–25.

18. Janssen I, Katzmarzyk PT, Ross R. Body mass index, waist circumference, and health risk: evidence in support of current National Institutes of Health guidelines. *Arch Intern Med* 2002;**162**(18):2074–9.

19. Blin O, Micallef J. Antipsychotic-associated weight gain and clinical outcome parameters. *J Clin Psychiatry* 2001;**62** Suppl. 7:11–21.

20. Wirshing DA, Pierre JM, Erhart SM, Boyd JA. Understanding the new and evolving profile of adverse drug effects in schizophrenia. *Psychiatr Clin North Am* 2003;**26**(1):165–90.

21. Travis MJ, Burns T, Dursun S, et al. Aripiprazole in schizophrenia: consensus guidelines. *Int J Clin Pract* 2005;**59** (4):485–95.

22. Lambert TJ. Switching to aripiprazole from olanzapine leads to weight loss in overweight people with schizophrenia or schizoaffective disorder. *Evid Based Ment Health* 2009;**12**(2):50.

23. Newcomer JW, Campos JA, Marcus RN, et al. A multicenter, randomized, double-blind study of the effects of aripiprazole in overweight subjects with schizophrenia or schizoaffective disorder switched from olanzapine. *J Clin Psychiatry* 2008;**69**(7):1046–56.

24. Bristol-Myers Squibb, Otsuka America Pharmaceutical. *Abilify (Aripiprazole) U.S. Full Prescribing Information.* Tokyo, Japan: Otsuka Pharmaceutical Co., Ltd.; 2008.

25. Henderson DC, Cagliero E, Gray C, et al. Clozapine, diabetes mellitus, weight gain, and lipid abnormalities: a five-year naturalistic study. *Am J Psychiatry* 2000;**157**(6):975–81.

26. Bobes J, Rejas J, Garcia-Garcia M, et al. Weight gain in patients with schizophrenia treated with risperidone, olanzapine, quetiapine or haloperidol: results of the EIRE study. *Schizophr Res* 2003;**62**(1–2):77–88.

27. McEvoy JP, Lieberman JA, Perkins DO, et al. Efficacy and tolerability of olanzapine, quetiapine, and risperidone in the treatment of early psychosis: a randomized, double-blind 52-week comparison. *Am J Psychiatry* 2007;**164** (7):1050–60.

28. Janssen-Ortho Inc. *Invega (Paliperidone) Canadian Product Monograph.* Toronto, Canada: Janssen-Ortho Inc.; 2008.

Ocular effects

Background

This chapter covers antipsychotic-related cataracts, corneal deposits, and pigmentary retinopathy. For information on blurred vision and glaucoma refer to Chapter 1.3 on anticholinergic effects.

Ocular changes associated with antipsychotic medications include lens deposits (deposition of pigmented or denatured protein on the lens surface), cataracts (clouding of the lens due to the coalescence and clumping of proteins), corneal deposits (impairment of vision by distorting light refraction), and pigmentary retinopathy (loss of photoreceptors on the retinal epithelium resulting in night blindness and loss of central vision) (Figure 1.10.1) [1–3].

The most prevalent adverse ocular effect of long-term antipsychotic treatment other than blurred vision (secondary to impaired accommodation, an anticholinergic effect) is the formation of cataracts. There are various types of cataracts (anterior and posterior subcapsular, cortical, and nuclear). In the general population, the most prevalent types of cataracts are cortical and nuclear. Anterior subcapsular cataracts, which are less visually impairing than other types, are the most common type associated with antipsychotic use, especially the phenothiazines, and are uncommon in the general population [4–6].

Risk factors associated with cataracts include age over 60 years, a family history, eye trauma, exposure to sunlight (UV-B rays), cigarette smoking, heavy alcohol consumption, and certain medications including corticosteroids, amiodarone, gold-based medications, allopurinol, miotics, and phenothiazine antipsychotics. Other commonly cited risk factors are less well established, including diabetes mellitus and hypertension [6–8].

Patients with schizophrenia have a higher rate of risk factors for cataract formation and appear to be at a significantly increased risk for some but not all types of cataracts. A case–control study that evaluated the rate of cataracts in people with schizophrenia ($n = 131$, 55 ± 12 years) compared with healthy controls ($n = 3271$, 59 ± 11 years) found a markedly higher rate of anterior subcapsular cataracts (26% vs. <0.2%) in the schizophrenia group. However, the rate of other cataracts was lower overall in this group (cortical 1.9% vs. 12%, $p < 0.002$; nuclear 1.9% vs. 10%, $p = 0.006$; and posterior subcapsular cataract 1.9% vs. 4%, $p = 0.22$) [4].

A study of younger patients (mean age: 35 years) with schizophrenia (as defined by the *Diagnostic and Statistical Manual of Mental Disorders*, 4th edn [DSM-IV]) living in a sunny equatorial climate also found a high rate (33%) of cataract formation, 77% of which were the anterior subcapsular type [9].

Not all studies have found a higher rate of cataracts associated with schizophrenia or antipsychotic use. However, a lower rate of eye examinations in people with chronic psychotic disorders may have contributed to these findings [10].

Agents of interest: cataracts

Second-generation antipsychotic agents

Clozapine

A single case report of pigmentary changes affecting the cornea and retina and the development of a stellate cataract in a 55-year-old woman treated long term

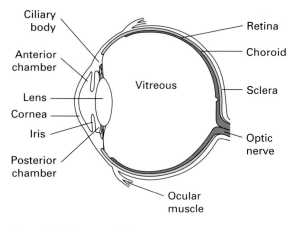

Figure 1.10.1 Anatomy of the eye.

with clozapine at high doses is the only evidence linking clozapine to cataracts. The causative role of clozapine is uncertain but is supported by ocular findings that are similar to those observed with chlorpromazine use [11].

Quetiapine

Quetiapine has been associated with an increased rate of cataract formation in dogs (beagles). The dose given was four times the maximum recommended dose in humans and was administered for 6–12 months. Cataract formation was not observed in similar studies performed in monkeys or other species [12–14].

Since quetiapine's approval in 1997, several million people have received quetiapine and fewer than 1/10 000 patients have reported lens abnormalities [14].

Phase II and III clinical trials reported a similar proportion of abnormal lens changes from baseline to final assessment for patients treated with quetiapine (2.8%), haloperidol (2.5%), and placebo (2.5%) [4].

Other second-generation antipsychotics

There are no reported causal associations between olanzapine, clozapine, risperidone, or ziprasidone and cataract formation [15].

No cases of cataracts have been located associated with aripiprazole or paliperidone, and their respective product monographs do not list this as an adverse effect [16,17].

First-generation antipsychotic agents

Phenothiazines (especially chlorpromazine and prochlorperazine, but also thioridazine, thiothixene, and trifluoperazine) have been associated with cataract formation. Risk may be dose related [15].

Chlorpromazine

Cases of lens and corneal deposition associated with chlorpromazine were reported soon after its release in the 1950s, and new cases continue to be reported [18–20].

Chlorpromazine can cause yellow–brown granules to be deposited under the anterior capsule, leading to lens opacities and anterior cataracts. Cataract incidence is associated with increased doses used for extended periods of time [3,15].

A cohort study of patients with schizophrenia (aged 30–85) taking chlorpromazine long term (>90 days) at doses ≥300 mg/day found a ninefold increase in risk of developing cataracts compared with the general population [10].

Vision disturbances due to pigment deposits in the cornea and lens are more commonly reported in patients receiving chlorpromazine at high doses (e.g. ≥800 mg/day for 2 years). However, cases of pigmentary deposits have also been documented at lower doses (e.g. 200 mg/day for 2 years) [15].

Other first-generation antipsychotics

Thioridazine has been reported to induce lenticular changes associated with cataract development, but this may be limited to long-term use of doses exceeding 800 mg/day [15].

A cohort study of patients with schizophrenia (aged 30–85) taking antipsychotics long term (>90 days) found that the risk of cataract development was increased fourfold with prochlorperazine [10].

Monitoring schedule for **ANTIPSYCHOTIC-INDUCED OCULAR CHANGES**

Monitoring includes assessment of pre-existing, new-onset, or changes in vision problems. At baseline, review the risk factors for cataract formation.

	Baseline	Weeks		Months					Long-term monitoring
		1	2	1	2	3	6	12	
Second-generation antipsychotics									
Aripiprazole	•								⊛ᵃ
Clozapine	•								⊛ᵃ
Olanzapine	•								⊛ᵃ
Paliperidone	•								⊛ᵃ
Quetiapine	•								⊛ᵃ
Risperidone	•								⊛ᵃ
Ziprasidone	•								⊛ᵃ
First-generation antipsychotics									
Chlorpromazine	•						•	•	⊛ ⑥ᵃ
Flupenthixol	•								⊛ᵃ
Fluphenazine	•						•	•	⊛ ⑥ᵃ
Haloperidol	•								⊛ᵃ
Loxapine	•								⊛ᵃ
Methotrimeprazine	•						•	•	⊛ ⑥ᵃ
Molindone	•								⊛ᵃ
Pericyazine	•								⊛ᵃ
Perphenazine	•						•	•	⊛ ⑥ᵃ
Pimozide	•								⊛ᵃ
Pipotiazine palmitate	•								⊛ᵃ
Thioridazine	•						•	•	⊛ ⑥ᵃ
Thiothixene	•								⊛ᵃ
Trifluoperazine	•						•	•	⊛ ⑥ᵃ
Zuclopenthixol	•								⊛ᵃ

• Monitor for adverse effect. ⊛ As clinically indicated. ⑥ Every 6 months.

ᵃ Screening for cataracts should begin at the age of 40 and continue every 5 years or more often, depending on patient age and the presence of multiple risk factors.

Agents of interest: pigmentary retinopathy

Second-generation antipsychotic agents

The very few reported cases, including the case of cataract and pigmentary retinopathy with clozapine described above, indicate that pigmentary retinopathy is very rare, if associated at all, with antipsychotic treatment.

First-generation antipsychotic agents

Thioridazine

Pigmentary changes of the retina have only been associated with thioridazine when used at exceptionally high doses. In one report, a 28-year-old woman was diagnosed with diffuse pigmentary retinopathy after receiving 3.2 g/day for 8 weeks. Dosages of 800 mg/day or less have not shown toxic retinal effects [21].

Monitoring

A vision history (e.g. recent changes in vision, presence of blurry vision) should be conducted for all patients starting antipsychotics.

Risk factors for cataract formation (see Background, p. 69) should be reviewed prior to initiating antipsychotic therapy.

Regular inquiries regarding vision problems are recommended for people taking chlorpromazine or other phenothiazines.

Blurred vision or other visual complaints by people taking antipsychotics long term, not explained otherwise, should lead to a formal eye examination for cataracts and other ocular changes.

Formal screening for cataracts is recommended in patients requiring long-term antipsychotic treatment when they reach the age of 40. This examination should be repeated every 5 years, or more frequently for patients presenting with several risk factors (e.g. treated with phenothiazines, smokers, heavy alcohol use, use of other medications associated with cataract formation) [22].

A slit-lamp eye examination is recommended if cataracts are suspected.

REFERENCES

1. Taylor F. Drugs affecting the eye. *Aust Fam Physician* 1985;**14**(8):744–5.
2. Sutton AL. *Eye Care Sourcebook: Basic Consumer Health Information About Eye Care and Eye Disorders*, 2nd edn. Detroit, MI: Omnigraphics; 2003.
3. Yanoff M, Duker JS. *Ophthalmology*, 2nd edn. London; St. Louis, MO: Mosby; 2004.
4. McCarty CA, Wood CA, Fu CL, et al. Schizophrenia, psychotropic medication, and cataract. *Ophthalmology* 1999;**106**(4):683–7.
5. Abraham AG, Condon NG, West Gower E. The new epidemiology of cataract. *Ophthalmol Clin North Am* 2006;**19**(4):415–25.
6. Hodge WG, Whitcher JP, Satariano W. Risk factors for age-related cataracts. *Epidemiol Rev* 1995;**17**(2):336–46.
7. Harper RA, Shock JP. Lens. In Riordan-Eva P, Whitcher JP, eds., *Vaughan & Asbury's General Ophthalmology*, 17th edn. USA: McGraw-Hill Companies, Inc.; 2008.
8. Marder SR, Essock SM, Miller AL, et al. Physical health monitoring of patients with schizophrenia. *Am J Psychiatry* 2004;**161**(8):1334–49.
9. Novais e Souza VB, de Moura Filho FJ, de Matos e Souza FG, et al. Cataract occurrence in patients treated with antipsychotic drugs. *Rev Bras Psiquiatr* 2008;**30**(3):222–6.
10. Ruigomez A, Garcia Rodriguez LA, Dev VJ, Arellano F, Raniwala J. Are schizophrenia or antipsychotic drugs a risk factor for cataracts? *Epidemiology* 2000;**11**(6):620–3.
11. Borovik AM, Bosch MM, Watson SL. Ocular pigmentation associated with clozapine. *Med J Aust* 2009;**190**(4):210–11.
12. AstraZeneca Canada Inc. *Seroquel XR (Quetiapine fumarate) Canadian Product Monograph*. Mississauga, ON: AstraZeneca Canada Inc.; 2009.
13. Stip E, Boisjoly H. Quetiapine: are we overreacting in our concern about cataracts (the beagle effect)? *Can J Psychiatry* 1999;**44**(5):503.
14. Nasrallah HA, Tandon R. Efficacy, safety, and tolerability of quetiapine in patients with schizophrenia. *J Clin Psychiatry* 2002;**63** Suppl. 13:12–20.
15. Shahzad S, Suleman MI, Shahab H, et al. Cataract occurrence with antipsychotic drugs. *Psychosomatics* 2002;**43**(5):354–9.

16. Bristol-Myers Squibb, Otsuka America Pharmaceutical. *Abilify (Aripiprazole) U.S. Full Prescribing Information.* Tokyo, Japan: Otsuka Pharmaceutical Co., Ltd.; 2008.

17. Janssen-Ortho Inc. *Invega (Paliperidone) Canadian Product Monograph.* Toronto, Canada: Janssen-Ortho Inc.; 2009.

18. Leung AT, Cheng AC, Chan WM, Lam DS. Chlorpromazine-induced refractile corneal deposits and cataract. *Arch Ophthalmol* 1999;**117**(12):1662–3.

19. Webber SK, Domniz Y, Sutton GL, Rogers CM, Lawless MA. Corneal deposition after high-dose chlorpromazine hydrochloride therapy. *Cornea* 2001;**20**(2):217–19.

20. Razeghinejad MR, Nowroozzadeh MH, Zamani M, Amini N. In vivo observations of chlorpromazine ocular deposits in a patient on long-term chlorpromazine therapy. *Clin Experiment Ophthalmol* 2008;**36**(6):560–3.

21. Shah GK, Auerbach DB, Augsburger JJ, Savino PJ. Acute thioridazine retinopathy. *Arch Ophthalmol* 1998;**116**(6):826–7.

22. Orlin SE. Cataracts. In American College of Physicians, ed., *ACP PIER & AHFS DI Essentials.* Philadelphia, PA: American College of Physicians; 2009.

Prolactin effects

Background

Prolactin belongs to the growth hormone family and is secreted by lactotroph cells in the anterior pituitary. Prolactin is primarily known for its functional roles in reproduction, pregnancy, and lactation, but has other functions, some relating to cytokine regulation and function [1,2].

Under normal conditions, dopamine secretion in the hypothalamus inhibits prolactin release. Antipsychotic-induced hyperprolactinemia results from dopaminergic blockade in the tubero-infundibular dopaminergic system of the hypothalamus. Due to its fenestrated capillary system, this region of the central nervous system does not have a blood–brain barrier. Various other medications (including selective serotonin reuptake inhibitors and tricyclic antidepressants, metoclopramide, domperidone, opiates, and methyldopa), some of which do not cross the blood–brain barrier, can cause mild to moderate elevations of prolactin [1,3,4].

The magnitude of hyperprolactinemia correlates strongly with dopamine D_2 receptor blockade potency. Due to marked variation among patients, prolactin level is a poor predictor of prolactin-related side effects. Hyperprolactinemia occurs more frequently in females than males, despite lower doses used in women [3,5].

Prolactin elevation occurs rapidly, usually within the first week, and is dose related. Little tolerance occurs to the hyperprolactinemic effects of antipsychotics. A reduction in prolactin level without a change in dose often signals non-adherence. A return to normal prolactin levels occurs rapidly upon discontinuation of treatment [3].

The primary clinical effects of hyperprolactinemia experienced by women and men in association with antipsychotic treatment are summarized in Table 1.11.1. Although less well established, other clinical effects may include reduced ejaculate volume and oligospermia in men as a result of hypogonadism. Other adverse effects of antipsychotics on sexual functioning not related to prolactin are summarized in Chapter 1.15 [3,6–10].

Osteoporosis, hypogonadism, and breast cancer have been associated with prolactinomas, in which prolactin levels can exceed 5000 ng/ml. To date, the research linking these complications with antipsychotic use is inadequate and no definitive conclusions can be made. Most studies suffer from limited sample size or important methodological flaws. No data are available to answer the question, "Does antipsychotic use increase the rate of bone fractures and related disability?" However, it is recommended that potent prolactin-elevating antipsychotics should be avoided in patients with known osteoporosis or a history of osteoporotic fractures. The results have been mixed among the few observational studies assessing the link with breast cancer, and more methodologically defensible studies are needed. However, at this time, it is recommended that prolactin-elevating antipsychotics be avoided in women with breast cancer [3,10–13].

The prevalence of galactorrhea associated with antipsychotic use in women has been reported from 10% to 90%, while it is rarely reported in men. Gynecomastia is a rare side effect in men with hyperprolactinemia, estimated to occur in 1–2%. Menstrual irregularities in

Table 1.11.1 Early-onset, reversible, clinical consequences of antipsychotic-induced hyperprolactinemia [10]

Women	Men
Galactorrhea	Galactorrhea
Gynecomastia	Gynecomastia
Oligomenorrhea	Reduced libido
Amenorrhea	Erectile dysfunction
Reduced libido	Ejaculatory dysfunction
Dyspareunia	
Vaginal dryness	

women with hyperprolactinemia are common, with rates between 48% and 88% reported in women taking either first-generation agents or risperidone. Rates of sexual dysfunction vary and depend on the study methods used to collect information on sexual functioning. Rates from 10% to 60% have been observed in patients taking antipsychotics; however, it is important to note that sexual dysfunction can result from factors other than hyperprolactinemia [10,11].

Agents of interest

Differences in research methodologies (e.g. different patient populations, length of follow-up, methods of inquiry, and case definitions) make it difficult to accurately and comparatively estimate the clinical impact of prolactin elevation among antipsychotics.

In general, the incidence of adverse effects attributable to hyperprolactinemia secondary to antipsychotic use has been researched inadequately.

Second-generation antipsychotic agents

Aripiprazole

Evidence from controlled trials indicates that aripiprazole does not cause an elevation in prolactin levels, likely explained by its partial agonist effect at dopamine D_2 receptors. A decrease in prolactin is common when switching from moderate- to high-potency dopamine antagonists to aripiprazole [10].

In a 4-week randomized controlled trial comparing aripiprazole and risperidone, hyperprolactinemia occurred in 91% of risperidone patients compared with 4.1% and 3.3% in aripiprazole patients treated with 20 mg/day and 30 mg/day, respectively [14].

In a post-hoc subanalysis of an 8-week, open-label study in outpatients with schizophrenia ($n = 269$), when patients were switched from risperidone or olanzapine to aripiprazole, mean prolactin levels decreased significantly by week 1 and remained lower over the 8-week study. Previously elevated prolactin levels in the risperidone group were reduced to normal range within 1 week [15].

Clozapine

Clozapine is generally not associated with significant rises in prolactin concentrations, and may instead be associated with reductions in prolactin upon switching from antipsychotics that cause hyperprolactinemia. If there is any prolactin elevation, it seems to be transient and asymptomatic [6,10,16].

Olanzapine

There is evidence that olanzapine may be associated with mild transient elevations of 2–20% in prolactin concentration [10,17,18].

Increases in prolactin occur within 1–8 weeks, but are rarely associated with clinical consequences [8,10].

Hyperprolactinemia occurs less frequently with olanzapine than with haloperidol and risperidone [8,17,19].

Paliperidone

Paliperidone is thought to have similar prolactin-elevating effects to risperidone [20].

In a 6-week, placebo-controlled trial in patients with acute schizophrenia, mean prolactin levels increased from normal ranges to abnormally high levels at end point in patients treated with paliperidone [21].

In a small study ($n = 25$) of patients taking oral risperidone, increased plasma prolactin levels correlated with 9-hydroxy-risperidone (paliperidone) levels and not with risperidone levels, suggesting that it is this metabolite that plays the predominant role in risperidone's effect on prolactin [22].

Quetiapine

Quetiapine is not associated with significant rises in prolactin concentrations. Rather, it is associated with reductions in prolactin upon switching from moderately to highly potent dopamine-blocking antipsychotics [10,23,24].

Risperidone

Evidence linking risperidone use with increased prolactin concentrations is considerable. Available data suggest that risperidone (and paliperidone) have the most potent hyperprolactinemic effect of all antipsychotics including haloperidol [6,8,16,17,19,25].

Elevated prolactin levels were seen in 74% and 91% of risperidone-treated patients in two large randomized controlled trials. In the CATIE trial (a large, double-blind, 18-month, randomized trial that compared olanzapine, risperidone, quetiapine, perphenazine, and ziprasidone therapy in patients that were previously on a variety of antipsychotics), only risperidone was associated with a mean increase in prolactin (13.8±1.4 ng/dl) [14,25,26].

Risperidone-associated increases in prolactin levels are dose-related, and concentrations tend to increase two-to threefold and are generally noticeable within the first few weeks of treatment [6,8,16].

The risk for clinical symptoms related to elevated prolactin levels is greatest with risperidone compared with other second-generation agents, and is similar to or greater than with moderately dosed haloperidol [27].

In one observational trial, the prevalence of hyperprolactinemia and abnormal menstrual cycles in women of reproductive age was 96% and 56% with risperidone ($n = 25$). With first-generation antipsychotics, the rates were 53% and 41%, respectively [28].

Ziprasidone

Treatment with ziprasidone has been associated with transient and mild increases in prolactin. Levels generally return to normal with chronic administration [10,29].

Some studies have shown no increase in prolactin levels or decreases from baseline prolactin levels [30–32].

First-generation antipsychotic agents

Evidence linking first-generation antipsychotic agent use with increased prolactin concentrations is considerable [6,10].

Many first-generation antipsychotic agents, such as chlorpromazine, haloperidol, and loxapine, have demonstrated the propensity to cause dose-dependent prolactin concentration elevations [6,10].

Although not typical, prolactin elevation associated with first-generation antipsychotics has been reported to be as high as seven times the upper limit of normal [6].

Haloperidol

Prolactin concentrations can rise to several times the baseline level with haloperidol use [17,23].

Significant increases in prolactin generally occur early, within the first few weeks of treatment, and can lead to hyperprolactinemia complications [8].

Risperidone causes similar or greater prolactin elevation and prolactin-related adverse effects than haloperidol [33,34].

Other first-generation antipsychotics

Other first-generation antipsychotics often cause hyperprolactinemia, the severity of which is dose dependent. This is most notable with the moderate- and high-potency agents including fluphenazine, flupenthixol, loxapine, perphenazine, pimozide, thiothixene, and trifluoperazine.

Monitoring

Prolactin

Prolactin should be measured at baseline (by obtaining a morning fasting plasma prolactin level) when starting a new course of a prolactin-elevating antipsychotic agent. Also, the presence and absence of possible hyperprolactinemia-related signs and symptoms should be documented at baseline and follow-up [35].

The upper limit of normal for prolactin (i.e. morning fasting prolactin) varies by age, gender, and pregnancy

Monitoring schedule for **ANTIPSYCHOTIC-INDUCED PROLACTIN EFFECTS**

Monitoring includes assessment of pre-existing, new-onset, and changes in prolactin-related clinical effects. A morning fasting prolactin level should be requested when indicated.

	Baseline	Weeks		Months					Long-term monitoring
		1	2	1	2	3	6	12	
Second-generation antipsychotics									
Aripiprazole	•								⊛
Clozapine	•								⊛
Olanzapine	•								⊛
Paliperidone	•			•		•	•	•	⊛ ⑥
Quetiapine	•								⊛
Risperidone	•			•		•	•	•	⊛ ⑥
Ziprasidone	•								⊛
First-generation antipsychotics									
Chlorpromazine	•			•		•	•	•	⊛ ⑥
Flupenthixol	•			•		•	•	•	⊛ ⑥
Fluphenazine	•			•		•	•	•	⊛ ⑥
Haloperidol	•			•		•	•	•	⊛ ⑥
Loxapine	•			•		•	•	•	⊛ ⑥
Methotrimeprazine	•			•		•	•	•	⊛ ⑥
Molindone	•			•		•	•	•	⊛ ⑥
Pericyazine	•			•		•	•	•	⊛ ⑥
Perphenazine	•			•		•	•	•	⊛ ⑥
Pimozide	•			•		•	•	•	⊛ ⑥
Pipotiazine palmitate	•			•		•	•	•	⊛ ⑥
Thioridazine	•			•		•	•	•	⊛ ⑥
Thiothixene	•			•		•	•	•	⊛ ⑥
Trifluoperazine	•			•		•	•	•	⊛ ⑥
Zuclopenthixol	•			•		•	•	•	⊛ ⑥

• Monitor for adverse effect. ⊛ As clinically indicated. ⑥ Every 6 months.

status. Prolactin levels peak between 4 am and 6 am. Factors that can elevate prolactin to keep in mind when interpreting prolactin results are exercise, sexual intercourse, meals, and acute stress (e.g. minor surgical procedures, injury). The half-life of prolactin is short (50 minutes), reducing the opportunity for these factors to affect a typical morning fasting prolactin measure. It should also be noted that the normal ranges quoted among laboratories vary to some extent [35].

Usual normal ranges for fasting adults are [36]:
- Non-pregnant women: 0–20 ng/ml (0–424 mIU/l].
- Pregnant women: ≤200 ng/ml (≤4240 mIU/l)
- Men: 0–15 ng/ml (0–318 mIU/l)

Clinical effects of hyperprolactinemia

Clinical effects associated with hyperprolactinemia typically do not manifest below 60 ng/ml (1272 mIU/l). However, there is marked individual variation making it difficult to identify any single clinically relevant plasma concentration threshold. Many women do not voluntarily inform their healthcare providers of side effects such as galactorrhea and amenorrhea. Consequently, clinical inquiry is paramount [6,33].

Patients taking antipsychotic medications with higher likelihood of causing hyperprolactinemia should be assessed for related clinical effects (see Table 1.11.1) every 6 months minimally.

The clinical consequences of hyperprolactinemia should be inquired about on a regular basis. Some of these adverse effects (e.g. sexual dysfunction) may have other causes that require consideration. A routine prolactin inquiry should include the following questions:

Have you experienced any changes in...	Men	Women
Sexual functioning:	Libido	Libido
	Erection	Lubrication
	Ejaculation	Orgasm
	Satisfaction	Satisfaction
	Pain	Pain
		Menstrual cycle
Breast tissue:		Lactation
		Tenderness

REFERENCES

1. Mancini T, Casanueva FF, Giustina A. Hyperprolactinemia and prolactinomas. *Endocrinol Metab Clin North Am* 2008;**37**(1):67–99, viii.
2. Ben-Jonathan N, Hugo ER, Brandebourg TD, LaPensee CR. Focus on prolactin as a metabolic hormone. *Trends Endocrinol Metab* 2006;**17**(3):110–16.
3. Baldessarini RJ, Tarazi FI. Pharmacotherapy of psychosis and mania. In Brunton LL, Lazo JS, Parker KL, eds., *Goodman & Gilman's The Pharmacological Basis of Therapeutics*, 11th edn. USA: McGraw-Hill; 2006.
4. Martin JH. *Neuroanatomy Text and Atlas*, 3rd edn. USA: McGraw-Hill Companies, Inc; 2003.
5. Kuruvilla A, Peedicayil J, Srikrishna G, Kuruvilla K, Kanagasabapathy AS. A study of serum prolactin levels in schizophrenia: comparison of males and females. *Clin Exp Pharmacol Physiol* 1992;**19**(9):603–6.
6. Hamner MB, Arana GW. Hyperprolactinaemia in antipsychotic-treated patients: guidelines for avoidance and management. *CNS Drugs* 1998;**10**(3):209–222.
7. Halbreich U, Kinon BJ, Gilmore JA, Kahn LS. Elevated prolactin levels in patients with schizophrenia: mechanisms and related adverse effects. *Psychoneuroendocrinology* 2003;**28** Suppl. 1:53–67.
8. Kinon BJ, Gilmore JA, Liu H, Halbreich UM. Hyperprolactinemia in response to antipsychotic drugs: characterization across comparative clinical trials. *Psychoneuroendocrinology* 2003;**28** Suppl. 2:69–82.
9. Wieck A, Haddad PM. Antipsychotic-induced hyperprolactinaemia in women: pathophysiology, severity and consequences. Selective literature review. *Br J Psychiatry* 2003;**182**:199–204.
10. Byerly M, Suppes T, Tran QV, Baker RA. Clinical implications of antipsychotic-induced hyperprolactinemia in patients with schizophrenia spectrum or bipolar spectrum disorders: recent developments and current perspectives. *J Clin Psychopharmacol* 2007;**27**(6):639–61.
11. Bostwick JR, Guthrie SK, Ellingrod VL. Antipsychotic-induced hyperprolactinemia. *Pharmacotherapy* 2009;**29**(1):64–73.
12. Wieck A, Haddad PM. Hyperprolactinemia. In Haddad PM, Dursun S, Deakin B, eds., *Adverse Syndromes and Psychiatric Drugs*. Oxford, UK: Oxford University Press; 2004.
13. Lehman AF, Lieberman JA, Dixon LB, et al. Practice guideline for the treatment of patients with schizophrenia, second edition. *Am J Psychiatry* 2004;**161**(2 Suppl.):1–56.

14. Potkin SG, Saha AR, Kujawa MJ, et al. Aripiprazole, an antipsychotic with a novel mechanism of action, and risperidone vs placebo in patients with schizophrenia and schizoaffective disorder. *Arch Gen Psychiatry* 2003;**60** (7):681–90.

15. Byerly MJ, Marcus RN, Tran QV, Eudicone JM, Whitehead R, Baker RA. Effects of aripiprazole on prolactin levels in subjects with schizophrenia during cross-titration with risperidone or olanzapine: analysis of a randomized, open-label study. *Schizophr Res* 2009;**107** (2–3):218–22.

16. Volavka J, Czobor P, Cooper TB, et al. Prolactin levels in schizophrenia and schizoaffective disorder patients treated with clozapine, olanzapine, risperidone, or haloperidol. *J Clin Psychiatry* 2004;**65**(1):57–61.

17. David SR, Taylor CC, Kinon BJ, Breier A. The effects of olanzapine, risperidone, and haloperidol on plasma prolactin levels in patients with schizophrenia. *Clin Ther* 2000;**22**(9):1085–96.

18. Crawford AM, Beasley CM, Jr, Tollefson GD. The acute and long-term effect of olanzapine compared with placebo and haloperidol on serum prolactin concentrations. *Schizophr Res* 1997;**26**(1):41–54.

19. Tran PV, Hamilton SH, Kuntz AJ, et al. Double-blind comparison of olanzapine versus risperidone in the treatment of schizophrenia and other psychotic disorders. *J Clin Psychopharmacol* 1997;**17**(5):407–18.

20. Janssen-Ortho Inc. *Invega (Paliperidone) Canadian Product Monograph*. Toronto, Canada: Janssen-Ortho Inc.; 2009.

21. Kane J, Canas F, Kramer M, et al. Treatment of schizophrenia with paliperidone extended-release tablets: a 6-week placebo-controlled trial. *Schizophr Res* 2007;**90** (1–3):147–61.

22. Knegtering R, Baselmans P, Castelein S, Bosker F, Bruggeman R, van den Bosch RJ. Predominant role of the 9-hydroxy metabolite of risperidone in elevating blood prolactin levels. *Am J Psychiatry* 2005;**162**(5):1010–12.

23. Atmaca M, Kuloglu M, Tezcan E, Canatan H, Gecici O. Quetiapine is not associated with increase in prolactin secretion in contrast to haloperidol. *Arch Med Res* 2002;**33**(6):562–5.

24. Copolov DL, Link CG, Kowalcyk B. A multicentre, double-blind, randomized comparison of quetiapine (ICI 204,636, 'seroquel') and haloperidol in schizophrenia. *Psychol Med* 2000;**30**(1):95–105.

25. Schooler N, Rabinowitz J, Davidson M, et al. Risperidone and haloperidol in first-episode psychosis: a long-term randomized trial. *Am J Psychiatry* 2005;**162**(5):947–53.

26. Lieberman JA, Stroup TS, McEvoy JP, et al. Effectiveness of antipsychotic drugs in patients with chronic schizophrenia. *N Engl J Med* 2005;**353**(12):1209–23.

27. Bezchlibnyk-Butler KZ, Jeffries JJ. *Clinical Handbook of Psychotropic Drugs*, 4th rev. edn. Toronto: Hogrefe & Huber Publishers; 1993.

28. Kinon BJ, Gilmore JA, Liu H, Halbreich UM. Prevalence of hyperprolactinemia in schizophrenic patients treated with conventional antipsychotic medications or risperidone. *Psychoneuroendocrinology* 2003;**28** Suppl. 2: 55–68.

29. Pfizer Canada Inc. *Zeldox (Ziprasidone hydrochloride) Canadian Product Monograph*. Quebec, Canada: Pfizer Canada Inc.; 2007.

30. Kane JM, Khanna S, Rajadhyaksha S, Giller E. Efficacy and tolerability of ziprasidone in patients with treatment-resistant schizophrenia. *Int Clin Psychopharmacol* 2006;**21**(1):21–8.

31. Weiden PJ, Daniel DG, Simpson G, Romano SJ. Improvement in indices of health status in outpatients with schizophrenia switched to ziprasidone. *J Clin Psychopharmacol* 2003;**23**(6):595–600.

32. Weiden PJ, Simpson GM, Potkin SG, O'Sullivan RL. Effectiveness of switching to ziprasidone for stable but symptomatic outpatients with schizophrenia. *J Clin Psychiatry* 2003;**64**(5):580–8.

33. Haddad PM, Wieck A. Antipsychotic-induced hyperprolactinaemia: mechanisms, clinical features and management. *Drugs* 2004;**64**(20):2291–314.

34. Kleinberg DL, Davis JM, de Coster R, Van Baelen B, Brecher M. Prolactin levels and adverse events in patients treated with risperidone. *J Clin Psychopharmacol* 1999;**19** (1):57–61.

35. Citrome L. Current guidelines and their recommendations for prolactin monitoring in psychosis. *J Psychopharmacol* 2008;**22**(2 Suppl.):90–7.

36. Kratz A, Ferraro M, Sluss PM, Lewandrowski KB. Case records of the Massachusetts General Hospital. Weekly clinicopathological exercises. Laboratory reference values. *N Engl J Med* 2004;**351**(15):1548–63.

QTc prolongation, arrhythmias, and sudden cardiac death

Background

The QT interval is the electrocardiographic representation of ventricular depolarization and repolarization. On a surface electrocardiogram (ECG), the QT interval initiates at the beginning of the QRS complex and concludes at the end of the T wave (Figure 1.12.1). Inter- and intra-patient variation exists, as the QT interval can be altered via various mechanisms, including diurnal effects, differences in autonomic tone, electrolyte abnormalities, and drugs [1].

The QT interval changes with heart rate; as the heart rate increases, the interval decreases. Measurement is thus corrected according to the heart rate, yielding a rate-corrected value (QTc). Accurately accounting for this effect of heart rate is especially important as many drugs that prolong the QT interval concomitantly alter heart rate [2].

Excessive prolongation of the QTc interval is associated with potentially fatal cardiac arrhythmias, most notably torsade de pointes, a ventricular arrhythmia that can lead rapidly to sudden cardiac death [1,3].

The QTc interval is considered normal, marginally prolonged, and abnormally prolonged in women if it is ≤450 ms, 451–470 ms, and >470 ms, and in men if it is ≤430 ms, 431–450 ms, >450 ms, respectively [4] (see Table 1.12.4 under Monitoring).

In people aged 55 years and older, marginally prolonged QTc intervals have been associated with a non-statistically significant 60% increase in risk of sudden cardiac death (hazard ratio [HR] = 1.6, 95% confidence interval [CI] 0.9–3.1) and abnormally prolonged QTc

intervals are associated with a 150% increased risk (HR = 2.5, 95% CI 1.3–4.7). However, it should be noted that these differences in risk were evident only after an extended follow-up time of 6.7 years on average. Unadjusted rates of sudden cardiac death at the average follow-up time for people with initially normal, marginal, and abnormal QTc intervals were 1.3%, 2.7%, and 4.8%, respectively [5].

There is general agreement that a drug-induced increase of ≥30 ms in QTc interval is concerning and that an increase of ≥60 ms or when the QTc interval exceeds 500 ms indicates that the risk is excessive [6].

Many but not all antipsychotic agents have been associated with QTc prolongation. However, the risk for sudden cardiac death appears to be increased among all commonly used first- and second-generation antipsychotics, presumably due to inhibition of the potassium IKr channel and prolongation of cardiac repolarization. This risk for sudden cardiac death appears to be approximately double that of the general population [3,7].

The incidence rate of sudden cardiac death with antipsychotics has been estimated at 2.9 events per 1000 patient-years. This is markedly higher than the risk of death due to agranulocytosis with clozapine, which is estimated at 0.2 per 1000 patient-years [8].

Collectively based on 17 randomized controlled trials involving elderly patients with dementia, the risk for death (from all causes) was found to be 1.6–1.7 times higher with second-generation antipsychotics compared with placebo. The leading causes of death were heart failure, sudden death, and pneumonia. The risk with first-generation agents is not thought to be lower [9,10].

Risk factors for arrhythmias related to QTc prolongation and sudden cardiac death are numerous (see Tables 1.12.1–1.12.3). Patients started on antipsychotic medications should be thoroughly evaluated for the presence of risk factors before and during treatment.

Table 1.12.1 Risk factors for arrhythmias [3,11,12]

Age
Drug interactions:
    Pharmacodynamic – drug synergism (Table 1.12.2)
    Pharmacokinetic – co-consumption with inhibitors of
        metabolism and elimination (Table 1.12.3)
Electrolyte imbalances (hypocalcemia, hypomagnesemia,
    hypokalemia)
Renal disease
Use of diuretics
Personal or family history of:
    Syncope (e.g. unexplained falls, dizziness, blackouts)
    Sudden unexplained death
    Arrhythmias
    Heart disease (e.g. angina, heart failure, ventricular
        hypertrophy)
    Bradycardia
    Congenital long QT syndrome
    Renal or hepatic impairment
Use of restraints
Substance abuse
Use of multiple QTc-prolonging agents (Table 1.12.2)

Drugs may cause QT prolongation directly or indirectly, for example when a second drug interferes with the clearance of another drug, which has a direct effect on cardiac electrophysiology. For an updated list of drugs likely to prolong the QTc interval or induce torsade de pointes, refer to the Arizona Center for Education and Research on Therapeutics at http://www.azcert.org/medical-pros/drug-lists/drug-lists.cfm.

Agents of interest

A two- to threefold increase in sudden cardiac death has been observed in large retrospective database studies focusing on first- and second-generation antipsychotic agents. Due to the rarity of this event, risk with individual drugs cannot be determined precisely. Epidemiological data support the probability that the risk of sudden cardiac death is dose related [7,13,14].

The international adverse experience with sertindole, which increased the QTc interval in relation to its dose and led to a disproportionately high number of sudden cardiac deaths, heightened the intensity of investigations assessing the effect of newer antipsychotics on the QTc interval. To a lesser extent, some older antipsychotics were also more closely assessed (e.g. thioridazine, mesoridazine, pimozide). However, the relationship of dose and plasma concentration on QTc interval for most older antipsychotics has not been investigated systematically. For these agents, most of what is known comes from spontaneous reporting. As

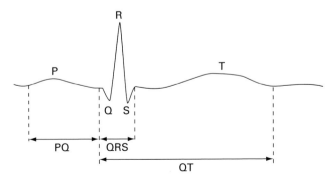

Figure 1.12.1 The electrocardiogram complex.

Table 1.12.2 Selected drugs known or suspected to prolong the QTc interval [1]

Very probable[a]	Probable[a]	Possible in high-risk patients[a]
Anti-arrhythmics	Antipsychotics	Anti-infectives
Amiodarone	Pimozide	Clarithromycin
Disopyramide	Ziprasidone	Erythromycin
Dofetilide		Gatifloxacin
Ibutilide		Pentamidine
Procainamide		Antipsychotics
Quinidine		Chlorpromazine
Sotalol		Haloperidol
Antipsychotics		Olanzapine
Thioridazine		Risperidone
		Antidepressants
		Amitriptyline
		Desipramine
		Imipramine
		Sertraline
		Venlafaxine
		Other
		Droperidol

[a] Categories are based on a survey of expert opinion. "Very probable" indicates that more than 50% of respondents stated they would always check ECG when starting this medication, "probable" indicates that 40–49% of respondents stated they would always check ECG when starting this medication, and "possible in high-risk patients" indicates that more than 40% of respondents stated they would always check ECG in high-risk patients.

such, the true rates of abnormally long QTc intervals among most first-generation agents are not precisely known [15,16].

Second-generation antipsychotic agents

The risk of sudden cardiac death appears similar when comparing first- and second-generation antipsychotic classes. Compared with people not taking antipsychotics, the risk is approximately doubled with either class. Individual differences in risk among antipsychotics have not been measured reliably [7].

Table 1.12.3 Selected drugs that slow the elimination of QTc-prolonging agents [1]

QTc-prolonging drugs	Drugs that inhibit the clearance of QTc-prolonging drugs
Anti-arrhythmics	
Disopyramide	Erythromycin
Dofetilide	Cimetidine, ketoconazole, megesterol, prochlorperazine, trimethoprim, verapamil, thiazide diuretics
Procainamide	Amiodarone, cimetidine, trimethoprim
Quinidine	Amiodarone, cimetidine, possibly erythromycin and verapamil
Antipsychotics	
Haloperidol	Fluoxetine, venlafaxine
Pimozide	Erythromycin
Thioridazine	Paroxetine
Antidepressants	
Amitriptyline	Cimetidine, fluconazole, fluoxetine, ritonavir
Desipramine	Venlafaxine
Anti-infectives	
Erythromycin	Ritonavir

The above list is not exhaustive. Refer to a comprehensive drug interactions reference for further information.

Aripiprazole

Aripiprazole does not appear to be associated with QTc prolongation [17].

Clozapine

One small study suggested that QTc >500 ms may be experienced in 3% of patients on clozapine. However, most data indicate that clozapine has little to no effect on the QT interval [18,19].

A large retrospective cohort study documented 19 sudden cardiac deaths among 4654 clozapine users (0.4%). The adjusted risk ratio for sudden cardiac death compared with non-antipsychotic users was 3.7 (95% CI 1.9–6.9) [7].

In retrospective studies and case reports, clozapine has been associated with the development of myocarditis and cardiomyopathy, some of which resulted in ECG changes, heart failure, and sudden cardiac death [20,21].

In Australia, Canada, the UK, and the USA, the Clozaril® national registries reported rates of myocarditis ranging from 5.0 per 100 000 to 97 per 100 000 patients treated [22].

Myocarditis occurred within the first 2 months of initiation of clozapine in 85% of cases. Based on an analysis of US data, one group estimated the incidence of fatal myocarditis during the first month of therapy to be 321 per 1 million person-years of treatment. This estimate greatly exceeds the expected rate of four cases of fatal myocarditis per million people treated for 1 year [23,24].

By early 2002, there were 178 cases of cardiomyopathy associated with clozapine in the Novartis international pharmacovigilance database, 32 of which were fatal. Onset was more gradual than with myocarditis, with 65% of cases being treated for more than 6 months [23].

Olanzapine

In an analysis of data from four randomized trials, the incidence of QTc ≥450 ms did not significantly differ from baseline [25].

In the CATIE trial, an 18-month, follow-up, randomized trial comparing five antipsychotics, none of the 231 eligible patients treated with olanzapine developed a prolonged QT interval [26].

Olanzapine ($n = 24$) had the smallest change in QTc interval, of 1.7 ms, of six antipsychotics studied in a randomized trial purposefully designed to assess QT changes at peak plasma concentration with and without coadministration of a cytochrome P450 enzyme inhibitor. Fluvoxamine, the inhibitor of olanzapine clearance, increased the peak olanzapine concentration by 77% but had no effect on QT [27].

Despite its relatively benign effect on QT, a large retrospective cohort study documented 75 sudden cardiac deaths among 27 257 olanzapine users (0.3%). The adjusted risk ratio for sudden cardiac death compared with non-antipsychotic users was 2.0 (95% CI 1.5–2.7) [7].

Paliperidone

Paliperidone is the active metabolite of risperidone. Its recent availability prevents an accurate assessment of its risk for adverse cardiac events. Its effect on the QT interval and its risk for sudden cardiac death are expected to be similar to but not in excess of that attributed to risperidone.

Quetiapine

Quetiapine ($n = 27$) was associated with a small mean increase in QTc interval of 5.7 ms when measured at peak plasma concentration. When taken with its metabolic inhibitor, ketoconazole, the plasma concentration of quetiapine increased fourfold, but there was no significant effect on QTc [27].

In the CATIE trial, 6 out of 214 patients (3%) taking quetiapine were found to have a prolonged QTc interval at some point during treatment [26].

A large retrospective cohort study documented 40 sudden cardiac deaths among 17 355 quetiapine users (0.2%). The adjusted risk ratio for sudden cardiac death compared with non-antipsychotic users was 1.9 (95% CI 1.3–2.7) [7].

Risperidone

At peak plasma concentrations, the mean increase in QTc associated with risperidone ($n = 20$) was 3.9 ms. Concurrent treatment with the enzyme inhibitor paroxetine more than doubled the concentration of risperidone; however, this was not associated with an increase in QTc interval in otherwise healthy patients with chronic psychotic disorders [27].

In the CATIE trial, 7 out of 218 patients (3%) taking risperidone were found to have a prolonged QTc interval at some point during treatment [26].

A large retrospective cohort study documented 85 sudden cardiac deaths among 24 589 risperidone users (0.3%). The adjusted risk ratio for sudden cardiac death compared with non-antipsychotic users was 2.9 (95% CI 2.3–3.8). These effects have been found to be dose related; the risk ratios for low, medium, and high doses were 1.9, 3.0, and 3.6 (all $p < 0.05$) [7].

Ziprasidone

The effect of ziprasidone on the QTc interval was compared with five other antipsychotics (haloperidol, olanzapine, quetiapine, risperidone, and thioridazine) in a randomized controlled trial that measured effects at peak plasma concentrations and in the presence of metabolic enzyme inhibition. Ziprasidone was found to increase the QTc interval by 15.9 ms. This was not changed in the presence of enzyme inhibition, despite a 39% increase in peak plasma concentration. This was approximately 9 ms longer than with haloperidol and 14 ms shorter than with thioridazine. QTc did not exceed 500 ms in any of the 31 patients allocated to ziprasidone [27].

In other short-term studies, ziprasidone has been shown to moderately increase the QT interval an average of 5–10 ms, compared with <3 ms with haloperidol and placebo. In clinical development, a QTc interval exceeding 500 ms was observed in 2 out of 3095 people (0.06%) taking ziprasidone compared with 1 out of 440 (0.23%) taking placebo [12].

When dosed at 320 mg/day, which is above the recommended maximum dose, the QTc interval increased an average of 22 ms [28].

Ziprasidone has been available in the USA since 2001 and has been used by over 1 million patients. Despite its ability to lengthen the QT interval, it has not been associated with an increase in the risk of sudden cardiac death [29].

First-generation antipsychotic agents

Chlorpromazine

From a large retrospective cohort study investigating the incidence of sudden cardiac death among patients receiving antipsychotics, chlorpromazine use was associated with a 3.6-fold (95% CI 1.4–9.7) increased risk of sudden cardiac death compared with the use of no antipsychotic agent [13].

Haloperidol

Evidence linking haloperidol to QTc prolongation, arrhythmias, and sudden death is significant [3].

Haloperidol has been reported to increase QTc by approximately 4–7 ms [3,27].

From a large retrospective cohort study investigating the incidence of sudden cardiac death among

antipsychotic users, haloperidol use was associated with an increased risk of sudden cardiac death 1.9 times (95% CI 1.1–3.3) greater than the risk associated with the use of no antipsychotic agent [13].

In a follow-up study using a similar design, there were 58 sudden cardiac deaths out of 21 728 patients (0.3%) treated with haloperidol, for an adjusted risk ratio of 1.6 (95% CI 1.2–2.2) when compared with non-antipsychotic users [7].

Perphenazine

In the CATIE trial, 2 out of 172 patients (1%) taking perphenazine were found to have a prolonged QTc interval at some point during treatment. The mean change in QTc was 1.4 ms [26].

Pimozide

Between 1971 and 1995, 16 deaths and 24 cases of serious cardiac events in patients prescribed pimozide were reported in the UK [3].

Thioridazine

Among all commonly used antipsychotics, thioridazine prolongs the QTc interval the most and is most strongly linked to an increased risk for sudden cardiac death. These effects have been found to be dose related [7,27].

The evidence linking thioridazine to QTc prolongation and sudden death is compelling and led to the withdrawal of thioridazine in several countries including Canada [3,30].

From a large prospective observational trial investigating the relationship between QTc prolongation and antipsychotic use, patients using thioridazine were 5.0 times more likely to develop QTc prolongation (>456 ms) compared with the use of no antipsychotic agent [30].

Thioridazine has been reported to increase QTc by approximately 30–35.0 ms [3,27].

From a case–control study and a large retrospective cohort study investigating the incidence of sudden cardiac death among antipsychotic users, thioridazine use was associated with an increased risk of sudden cardiac death 3.0–5.5 times greater than the risk associated with the use of no antipsychotic agent [13,31].

In a follow-up study using a similar design, there were 65 sudden cardiac deaths out of 15 715 patients (0.4%) treated with thioridazine, for an adjusted risk ratio of 3.2 (95% CI 2.4–4.2) when compared with non-antipsychotic users [7].

Thiothixene

From a large retrospective cohort study investigating the incidence of sudden cardiac death among antipsychotic users, thiothixene use was associated with an increased risk of sudden cardiac death 4.2 times (95% CI 2.0–8.9) greater than the risk associated with the use of no antipsychotic agent [13].

Monitoring

In the absence of sensitive markers predicting arrhythmias and/or sudden cardiac death, the screening and monitoring of patients taking antipsychotics for these outcomes can be a vexing issue for clinicians. Determining who should receive an ECG or a more involved medical work-up before starting an antipsychotic requires consideration of the patient's risk factors and the antipsychotic selected and will mostly be determined by the clinician's judgement and the patient's preference.

First and foremost, the need for the antipsychotic should be considered thoroughly, especially for vulnerable patients (e.g. pediatrics, elderly) for whom the benefits are not clearly established (e.g. dementia) [8].

Prior to initiating antipsychotic treatment, it is recommended that all patients be assessed for risk factors associated with QTc prolongation and sudden cardiac death (see Tables 1.12.1–1.12.3) and these risk factors should also be identified throughout the treatment process. In particular, a personal or family history of syncope or a family history of sudden unexplained death should be investigated as potential indicators of congenital long QT syndrome [12].

In addition, patients should be informed of the common and serious hazards of taking antipsychotic medications, including the risk of developing a potentially fatal adverse effect, including an arrhythmia. The patient, or substitute decision-maker, can then contribute meaningfully to the decision of what should be monitored, how, and by whom.

An ECG tracing at baseline and in follow-up should be considered when one or more risk factors are present, when it is deemed necessary based on the physician's judgement, or when the patient or caregiver requests it. Table 1.12.4 provides thresholds for clinical interpretation of the QTc interval.

Although the risk of a serious arrhythmia or sudden death is rare even in the presence of risk factors, screening and monitoring efforts should be escalated for patients with known risk factors (see Table 1.12.1).

Age is an important risk factor to consider. In their assessment of QTc interval and risk of sudden cardiac death, Straus and colleagues noted that the risk of sudden death in the 55–68-year-old group with abnormally prolonged QTc intervals was eight times higher than those with normal QTc intervals. This indirect evidence suggests that antipsychotic-induced QT prolongation may be particularly concerning in older adults [5].

For clozapine's cardiotoxic risk, age does not appear to be associated with risk. Most cases of myocarditis and cardiomyopathy have occurred in patients under 50 years of age [23].

Pre-existing cardiovascular disease is also an important risk factor, in which risk is stratified by severity. For every 10 000 patient-years of follow-up, the numbers of sudden deaths attributable to antipsychotic use in people with no, mild, moderate, and severe pre-existing cardiovascular disease have been estimated to be 4, 21, 23, and 367, respectively, with risk ratios ranging from 1.6 ($p = 0.12$) to 3.53 ($p = 0.001$) [13].

Table 1.12.4 Standard QTc interval thresholds [4,6]

	Female (ms)	Male (ms)
Normal	≤450	≤430
Borderline	451–470	431–450
Prolonged	>470	>450
Significantly increased risk for arrhythmia	Change from baseline ≥60 ms or QTc >500 ms	

Monitoring schedule for QTc PROLONGATION, OTHER ARRHYTHMIAS, AND RISK OF SUDDEN CARDIAC DEATH

At minimum, monitoring includes assessment of risk factors at baseline and follow-up as well as clinical assessment of the development of signs and symptoms consistent with cardiac arrhythmias or other toxicities; ECGs can be used, based on the clinician's judgement and patient's preference, to augment clinical monitoring.

	Baseline	Weeks 1	Weeks 2	Months 1	Months 2	Months 3	Months 6	Months 12	Long-term monitoring
Second-generation antipsychotics									
Aripiprazole	•		•	•		•			(★)
Clozapine	•		•	•		•			(★)
Olanzapine	•		•	•		•			(★)
Paliperidone	•		•	•		•			(★)
Quetiapine	•		•	•		•			(★)
Risperidone	•		•	•		•			(★)
Ziprasidone	•		•	•		•			(★)
First-generation antipsychotics									
Chlorpromazine	•		•	•		•			(★)
Flupenthixol	•		•	•		•			(★)
Fluphenazine	•		•	•		•			(★)
Haloperidol	•		•	•		•			(★)
Loxapine	•		•	•		•			(★)
Methotrimeprazine	•		•	•		•			(★)
Molindone	•		•	•		•			(★)
Pericyazine	•		•	•		•			(★)
Perphenazine	•		•	•		•			(★)
Pimozide	•		•	•		•			(★)
Pipotiazine palmitate	•		•	•		•			(★)
Thioridazine	•		•	•		•			(★)
Thiothixene	•		•	•		•			(★)
Trifluoperazine	•		•	•		•			(★)
Zuclopenthixol	•		•	•		•			(★)

• Monitor for adverse effect. (★) As clinically indicated.

High doses of antipsychotics have been associated with an increase in risk. If high doses are being used, vitals and risk factors should be assessed more frequently. Again, the use and frequency of ECGs needs to be discussed between the patient and clinician [7,13].

When possible, the QTc interval should be measured during peak plasma concentrations of a QTc-prolonging medication [1].

It is important to keep in mind that a normal ECG should not be interpreted to mean no risk of arrhythmia. It merely indicates that there were no abnormalities when the ECG was conducted. Follow-up assessment needs to continually evaluate the presence or worsening of factors that risk QT prolongation or other arrhythmias associated with sudden cardiac death [12].

Whether or not ECG monitoring is applied, the following clinical signs and symptoms should be assessed as part of routine clinical practice of patients taking antipsychotics:

- Vital sign measures (see Chapter 1.21)
- Recent history of fainting spells or blackouts
- Racing heart/tachycardia
- Pounding heart/irregular heart rate
- Shortness of breath/increased respiratory rate
- Peripheral edema
- Fatigue
- Low blood pressure, dizziness/hypotension

REFERENCES

1. Al-Khatib SM, LaPointe NM, Kramer JM, Califf RM. What clinicians should know about the QT interval. *JAMA* 2003;**289**(16):2120–7.
2. Goldfrank LR, Flomenbaum N. *Goldfrank's Toxicologic Emergencies*, 8th edn. New York: McGraw-Hill, Medical Publishing Division; 2006.
3. Haddad PM, Anderson IM. Antipsychotic-related QTc prolongation, torsade de pointes and sudden death. *Drugs* 2002;**62**(11):1649–71.
4. Committee for Proprietary Medicinal Products. *Points to Consider: the Assessment of the Potential for QT Interval Prolongation by Non-cardiovascular Medicinal Products*. London, UK: The European Agency for the Evaluation of Medicinal Products: Human Medicines Evaluation Unit; 1997.
5. Straus SM, Kors JA, De Bruin ML, et al. Prolonged QTc interval and risk of sudden cardiac death in a population of older adults. *J Am Coll Cardiol* 2006;**47**(2):362–7.
6. Zareba W, Lin DA. Antipsychotic drugs and QT interval prolongation. *Psychiatr Q* 2003;**74**(3):291–306.
7. Ray WA, Chung CP, Murray KT, Hall K, Stein CM. Atypical antipsychotic drugs and the risk of sudden cardiac death. *N Engl J Med* 2009;**360**(3):225–35.
8. Schneeweiss S, Avorn J. Antipsychotic agents and sudden cardiac death – how should we manage the risk? *N Engl J Med* 2009;**360**(3):294–6.
9. US Food and Drug Administration. *Public Health Advisory: Deaths with Antipsychotics in Elderly Patients with Behavioral Disturbances*. US Food and Drug Administration; 2009.
10. Wang PS, Schneeweiss S, Avorn J, et al. Risk of death in elderly users of conventional vs. atypical antipsychotic medications. *N Engl J Med* 2005;**353**(22):2335–41.
11. Calderone V, Testai L, Martinotti E, Del Tacca M, Breschi MC. Drug-induced block of cardiac HERG potassium channels and development of torsade de pointes arrhythmias: the case of antipsychotics. *J Pharm Pharmacol* 2005;**57**(2):151–61.
12. Kutcher S, Brooks SJ, Gardner DM, et al. Expert Canadian consensus suggestions on the rational, clinical use of ziprasidone in the treatment of schizophrenia and related psychotic disorders. *Neuropsychiatr Dis Treat* 2005;**1**(2):89–108.
13. Ray WA, Meredith S, Thapa PB, Meador KG, Hall K, Murray KT. Antipsychotics and the risk of sudden cardiac death. *Arch Gen Psychiatry* 2001;**58**(12):1161–7.
14. Straus SM, Bleumink GS, Dieleman JP, et al. Antipsychotics and the risk of sudden cardiac death. *Arch Intern Med* 2004;**164**(12):1293–7.
15. Liu BA, Juurlink DN. Drugs and the QT interval – caveat doctor. *N Engl J Med* 2004;**351**(11):1053–6.
16. Glassman AH, Bigger JT, Jr. Antipsychotic drugs: prolonged QTc interval, torsade de pointes, and sudden death. *Am J Psychiatry* 2001;**158**(11):1774–82.
17. Travis MJ, Burns T, Dursun S, et al. Aripiprazole in schizophrenia: consensus guidelines. *Int J Clin Pract* 2005;**59**(4):485–95.
18. Kang UG, Kwon JS, Ahn YM, et al. Electrocardiographic abnormalities in patients treated with clozapine. *J Clin Psychiatry* 2000;**61**(6):441–6.
19. Warner B, Hoffmann P. Investigation of the potential of clozapine to cause torsade de pointes. *Adverse Drug React Toxicol Rev* 2002;**21**(4):189–203.

20. Hoehns JD, Fouts MM, Kelly MW, Tu KB. Sudden cardiac death with clozapine and sertraline combination. *Ann Pharmacother* 2001;**35**(7–8):862–6.

21. Killian JG, Kerr K, Lawrence C, Celermajer DS. Myocarditis and cardiomyopathy associated with clozapine. *Lancet* 1999;**354**(9193):1841–5.

22. Novartis Pharmaceuticals Corporation. *Important Drug Warning: Clozaril (Clozapine)*. East Hanover, NJ: Novartis Pharmaceuticals Corp.; 2002.

23. Novartis Pharmaceuticals Canada Inc. *Important Drug Safety Information: Association of Clozaril (Clozapine) with Cardiovascular Toxicity*. Dorval, QC: Novartis Pharmaceuticals Canada Inc.; 2002.

24. La Grenade L, Graham D, Trontell A. Myocarditis and cardiomyopathy associated with clozapine use in the United States. *N Engl J Med* 2001;**345**(3):224–5.

25. Czekalla J, Beasley CM, Jr, Dellva MA, Berg PH, Grundy S. Analysis of the QTc interval during olanzapine treatment of patients with schizophrenia and related psychosis. *J Clin Psychiatry* 2001;**62**(3):191–8.

26. Lieberman JA, Stroup TS, McEvoy JP, et al. Effectiveness of antipsychotic drugs in patients with chronic schizophrenia. *N Engl J Med* 2005;**353**(12):1209–23.

27. Harrigan EP, Miceli JJ, Anziano R, et al. A randomized evaluation of the effects of six antipsychotic agents on QTc, in the absence and presence of metabolic inhibition. *J Clin Psychopharmacol* 2004;**24**(1):62–9.

28. Miceli J, Shiovitz T, Swift R, Anziano R, Tensfeldt T. High-dose ziprasidone is associated with marginal additional QTc increase (abstract of poster). In *American Psychiatric Association 156th Annual Meeting*; May 17–22, 2003; San Francisco, CA.

29. Glassman AH. Schizophrenia, antipsychotic drugs, and cardiovascular disease. *J Clin Psychiatry* 2005;**66** Suppl. 6: 5–10.

30. Reilly JG, Ayis SA, Ferrier IN, Jones SJ, Thomas SH. QTc-interval abnormalities and psychotropic drug therapy in psychiatric patients. *Lancet* 2000;**355**(9209):1048–52.

31. Reilly JG, Ayis SA, Ferrier IN, Jones SJ, Thomas SH. Thioridazine and sudden unexplained death in psychiatric in-patients. *Br J Psychiatry* 2002;**180**:515–22.

Sedation and sleep disturbances

Background

Antipsychotics are used commonly in the management of patients with long-standing sleep problems. The altered sleep pattern may be related to the primary condition being treated (e.g. psychoses and affective disorders) or may be due to secondary factors such as poor sleep hygiene or the use of substances that can adversely affect sleep (e.g. psychostimulants, antidepressants, alcohol, and substance abuse). They can also be the cause of excessive sedation and other sleep problems [1,2].

Sleep consists of rapid eye movement (REM) and non-REM types. There are three stages of non-REM sleep, N1 (somnolence or drowsy sleep), N2 (lack of conscious awareness), and N3 (deep, delta, or slow-wave sleep). Normally, 20–25% of total sleep time is REM sleep and is associated with muscular atonia and vivid dreams [3].

In schizophrenia, common sleep disturbances include sleep-onset delay and maintenance sleep problems. In polysomnography studies, this is observed as markedly increased N2 sleep latency. Total sleep time and overall sleep efficiency are typically reduced. In one study, sleep efficiency was 72% in patients with schizophrenia previously treated with antipsychotics, 78% in never-treated patients, and 95% in the unaffected control group. Slow-wave sleep (N3) is reduced in schizophrenia. Increases in slow-wave sleep time are associated with improved memory consolidation, as is an increase in the density of sleep spindles. Olanzapine has been found to increase slow-wave sleep time but reduce the density of sleep spindles. These counteracting effects may explain the lack of effect of olanzapine on memory performance found in one study [4–6].

Although antipsychotics can improve sleep problems, with some of them commonly being used for this reason, they can also cause sedation and sleep problems. Antipsychotics can cause daytime sedation and can adversely alter the sleep–wake cycle, depending on the antipsychotic used and its dosing regimen. They have been associated with restless leg syndrome, periodic limb movement disorder, and somnambulism. Sleep apnea is most strongly associated with obesity, which is common in people with schizophrenia and is promoted by several commonly used antipsychotics. Antipsychotic-induced sedation can compromise patient evaluation, for example in the cognitive assessment of nursing home patients. There is also concern that the use of sedating antipsychotics can impair a return of functioning. It should also be noted that drug-induced sedation is associated with an increased risk of falls, traffic and other accidents, and reduced work productivity [2,7,8].

Patient surveys have indicated that excessive sedation caused by antipsychotics is a particularly bothersome adverse effect, one that is often underestimated by health providers. In the CATIE trial (an 18-month, follow-up, randomized trial comparing five antipsychotics), excessive sedation was reported as the third most common adverse effect leading to treatment discontinuation [9,10].

Medication-induced sedation is thought to occur as a result of blockade of various central receptors, including histamine H_1, α_1 adrenergic, and muscarinic M_1 receptors. Also, it is important to note that blockade of dopamine D_2 receptors, especially when receptor occupancy rates are high, can lead to a loss of spontaneity and impulse inhibition, which may be experienced

Table 1.13.1 Receptor-binding affinities of antipsychotics[a] [12–14]

	Dopamine D_2	Histamine H_1	Adrenergic α_1	Muscarinic	Serotonin 5-HT_{2a}	Serotonin 5-HT_{2c}
Aripiprazole	0.34	61	57	>10 000	3.4	–
Chlorpromazine	19	9.1	0.6	60	1.4	–
Clozapine	180	2.7	9	7.5	1.6	4.8
Flupenthixol	–	–	–	–	–	–
Fluphenazine	0.80	21	9.0	2000	19	–
Haloperidol	4	1890	6.2	>20 000	36	4700
Loxapine	71	5	28	62	1.7	–
Methotrimeprazine	–	–	–	–	–	–
Molindone	125	>10 000	2500	>20 000	5000	–
Olanzapine	11	7.1	19	1.9	4	4.1
Paliperidone	2.8	3.4	10.1	8800	1.2	48
Pericyazine	–	–	–	–	–	–
Perphenazine	1.40	8.3	10	1500	5.60	–
Pimozide	2.5	–	–	–	13	570
Pipotiazine palmitate	–	–	–	–	–	–
Quetiapine	160	11	62	120	294	3500
Risperidone	3.3	59	2	>10 000	0.16	32
Thioridazine	2.3	1.9	1.1	10	41	–
Thiothixene (*cis*)	0.4	6	11	2500	130	–
Trifluoperazine	2.6	62	28	670	–	–
Ziprasidone	0.42	47	10	>10 000	0.42	0.9
Zuclopenthixol	–	–	–	–	–	–

[a] Data are K_i values (nM) determined by competition with radioligands for binding to the indicated receptors. Lower values indicate higher affinities.

subjectively as tiredness. Antagonism of histamine H_1 and serotonin 5-HT_{2c} receptors, common to several antipsychotics, are also associated with weight gain, which can lead to or exacerbate sleep apnea and related daytime drowsiness. Receptor affinity estimates are provided in Table 1.13.1 [2,11,12].

The experience of sedation or insomnia can relate to the types of medications used when making treatment switches. For example, when switching between an antipsychotic with prominent effects to one that is noticeably less sedating, the patient may describe insomnia. Planning for this in advance can help to reduce this subjectively experienced adverse effect.

The effects of several antipsychotics on sleep architecture have been evaluated in polysomnographic sleep studies, the findings of which are summarized in Table 1.13.2.

Agents of interest

Caution should be exercised when interpreting the findings of antipsychotic studies reporting rates of sedation, somnolence, insomnia, and other sleep-related adverse events. In general, clinical trials do not report rates based on their inferred causality. A participant who describes morning somnolence during a clinical trial who has experienced the same type of somnolence before entering the trial will be counted no differently than a person who develops morning somnolence for

Table 1.13.2 Polysomnographic observed sleep effects of antipsychotics[a] [2,4,15]

	Tmax (h)	Half-life (h)	Total sleep time	REM suppression	Increases slow-wave sleep	Shortens sleep-onset latency	Decreases awakenings and wake time
Clozapine	3	16	+ + +	0	+	+	+ + +
Haloperidol	4–6	12–36	+ + +	+	+ +	+ + +	+ + +
Olanzapine	5	30	+ + +	0	+ + +	+	+ + +
Paliperidone	24	23	++	0	0	++	++
Quetiapine (XR)	1 [6]	7	+ + +	+ +	0	+ + +	+ + +
Risperidone	1	3–20	+	+ + +	+ + +	+	+ +
Thiothixene	2–4	34	+ + +	+	+ +	+ + +	+ + +
Ziprasidone	5	4–10	+ + +	+ + +	+ + +	+	+ + +

[a] Polysomnographic studies are available for several but not all antipsychotics and quality varies among the available studies. Head-to-head comparisons are generally not available, thereby limiting the comparability of sleep effects among antipsychotics. Moreover, differences in participant characteristics, study methods, and dosing regimens further limit the utility of the observations [4].

the first time shortly after starting the study treatment. Also, it is important to note that adverse event rates do not adequately characterize the problem. Missing are the details of intensity, frequency, duration, and consequences of the problem. Moreover, rates vary depending on how the adverse event was assessed. Trials will report higher rates when specific adverse events are queried compared with trials documenting only those spontaneously reported by participants. This and other factors may explain the large variation in rates of sedation or somnolence observed in placebo groups. These limitations need to be considered when interpreting the information provided in Table 1.13.3.

Second-generation antipsychotic agents

Provided below is a summary of the main findings of sedation and insomnia rates from head-to-head randomized controlled trials of antipsychotics in schizophrenia. Other information regarding antipsychotic-related sleep problems is also provided.

Aripiprazole

In two comparative studies with olanzapine, aripiprazole was associated with less somnolence (8% vs. 15–23%) and possibly more insomnia (27–32% vs. 17–30%) [17,18].

When compared with ziprasidone, aripiprazole revealed a similar rate of insomnia (7.0% vs. 6.4%) but a lower rate of somnolence with aripiprazole (13% vs. 26%), whereas, when compared with haloperidol, the rates of insomnia (22% vs. 20%) and somnolence (5% vs. 7%) were similar [19,20].

Clozapine

Clozapine has been found to increase N2 sleep, total sleep time, and sleep efficiency. It may reduce slow-wave sleep but does not appear to affect REM sleep [4].

Rates of sedation with clozapine are generally higher than with other antipsychotics. In comparison with risperidone, rates are approximately 40% with clozapine and 25% with risperidone. Hypersomnia was more common with clozapine (24%) compared with olanzapine (13%) in one study [21].

In phase 2E of the CATIE trial, hypersomnia (sleepiness) was most common with clozapine (45%) compared with quetiapine (33%), olanzapine (32%), and risperidone (25%). Insomnia was reported to occur in the reverse order: risperidone 31%, olanzapine 16%, quetiapine 13%, and clozapine 4% [22].

Case reports have implicated clozapine as an apparently rare cause of cataplexy as well as restless leg syndrome [23–26].

Table 1.13.3 Rates of insomnia and sedation among antipsychotics[a] [2,16]

	Insomnia/disturbed sleep (%)	Somnolence (%)
Aripiprazole	24	8–12
Chlorpromazine	–	33
Clozapine	4	52
Haloperidol	25	23
Olanzapine	18	29
Paliperidone	12	10
Quetiapine	9	16
Risperidone	17	30
Thioridazine	23	35–57
Ziprasidone	9	16

[a] With the exception of paliperidone, data presented are adapted from [2], which used data available in meta-analyses to estimate the rates of adverse events.

Olanzapine

In the CATIE trial, olanzapine had the lowest rate of insomnia (16%) compared with ziprasidone (30%), perphenazine (25%), risperidone (24%), and quetiapine (18%). It shared the highest rate of hypersomnia (sleepiness) with quetiapine (31%), which was marginally higher than with risperidone (28%) and perphenazine (28%) and distinct from ziprasidone (24%) [10].

Case reports indicate that olanzapine can be a cause of somnambulism, sometimes involving night-time gorging, as well as restless leg syndrome [27–32].

Paliperidone

A single trial of 6 days' duration comparing paliperidone and risperidone ($n = 113$) suggested that paliperidone is more sedating than its parent drug, risperidone. It reported sedation rates of 4% vs. 0% and insomnia rates of 8% and 18% for paliperidone and risperidone, respectively. Paliperidone differs from risperidone (which is metabolized extensively to paliperidone) in that it has significantly higher affinity for blocking histamine receptors, which may account for its apparently greater sedative effect than risperidone [12,16].

In comparisons with olanzapine, the rates of sedation and insomnia were 9% vs. 19% and 13% vs. 12% with paliperidone and olanzapine, respectively [16].

The 2-week rates of somnolence with paliperidone, when compared with quetiapine and placebo in the management of inpatients with recent exacerbation of schizophrenia, were 9%, 12%, and 1%, respectively. Insomnia was reported at similar rates among the three groups (10%, 9%, and 11%) [33].

In other placebo-controlled trials, the rates of sedation were 10% and 7% with paliperidone and placebo, respectively. Insomnia was reported in both groups at a rate of 12% [16].

Quetiapine

Quetiapine has been found to increase total sleep time, increase N2 sleep, reduce sleep latency, reduce awakenings, and improve subjective sleep quality in healthy persons and in patients with bipolar depression [2,34,35].

In the CATIE trial, quetiapine had a relatively low rate of insomnia (18%) compared with ziprasidone (30%), perphenazine (25%), risperidone (24%) and olanzapine (16%), and a relatively high rate of hypersomnia (sleepiness) (31%) compared with the other agents (31%, 28%, 28%, and 24%, respectively). In an earlier comparison with risperidone, the higher rate of sedation with quetiapine was more distinct (31% vs. 15%). For other details comparing quetiapine and risperidone, refer to the section on risperidone below [10,36].

Quetiapine has been implicated in several cases of restless leg syndrome. In addition, two cases of somnambulism have been reported with quetiapine involving male patients of 52 and 18 years at doses of ≥200 mg/day and 400 mg/day, respectively [37–39].

Risperidone

In the CATIE trial, risperidone (24%) had an intermediate rate of insomnia compared with ziprasidone (30%), perphenazine (25%), quetiapine (18%), and olanzapine (16%). It was similarly intermediate in the rate of hypersomnia (sleepiness) (28%) compared with olanzapine (31%), quetiapine (31%), perphenazine (28%), and ziprasidone (24%) [10].

In an 8-week study comparing risperidone and quetiapine ($n = 673$), more specific details regarding the sedating effects of each treatment were provided. Somnolence, which occurred at rates of 19.7% and 26.3%, was rated as mild by 65% and 70%, respectively. The mean durations of somnolence were similar at 9.6 and 10.5 days with risperidone and quetiapine. Somnolence led to two patients stopping quetiapine and one patient stopping risperidone [40].

Reports have implicated risperidone as a rare cause of restless leg syndrome, somnambulism involving night-time gorging, and night terrors [41–43].

Ziprasidone

Sedation occurs more often with olanzapine (30%) and quetiapine (29%) compared with ziprasidone (20%). In comparisons involving risperidone, the rates of sedation were 24% with risperidone and 20% with ziprasidone [44].

In the CATIE trial, ziprasidone had the highest rate of insomnia (30%) compared with perphenazine (25%), risperidone (24%), quetiapine (18%), and olanzapine (16%) [10].

Insomnia is a well-described adverse effect early in the treatment course of ziprasidone and frequently leads to premature discontinuation.

First-generation antipsychotic agents

Provided below is a general overview of the sedative effects among the first-generation antipsychotics. Also provided is a summary of the main findings of sedation and insomnia rates from head-to-head randomized controlled trials. Other information regarding antipsychotic-related sleep problems is also provided.

Polysomnographic studies have been conducted involving patients taking haloperidol, thiothixene, and flupenthixol, and indicate that these agents and possibly other first-generation agents have little effect on sleep architecture. These antipsychotics were found to improve sleep efficiency, reduce N2 sleep latency,

and increase total sleep time. There appears to be little effect on REM sleep other than an increase in REM sleep latency [4].

While sedation is a side effect of most if not all first-generation antipsychotics, the intensity of this effect is dependent on agent and dose. In general, lower-potency agents (sometimes referred to as high-milligram, low-potency antipsychotics), such as chlorpromazine, thioridazine, methotrimeprazine, and mesoridazine, cause the most sedation [12–14].

Chlorpromazine

Among the several small studies comparing chlorpromazine and haloperidol, the rates of sedation were 34% and 24%, respectively. Chlorpromazine and clozapine have been compared in numerous trials, which indicate that clozapine is more sedating (37% vs. 30%). Numerous placebo-controlled trials were completed in the 1960s and 1970s. Sedation with chlorpromazine was 33% compared with 13% with placebo [45–47].

Haloperidol

As noted above, haloperidol causes sedation less often than chlorpromazine (25% vs. 34%). Rates of sedation appear similar between haloperidol and risperidone (26% vs. 29%), whereas insomnia occurred slightly more often with haloperidol (22% vs. 17%). Approximately 350 patients were evaluated in placebo-controlled studies. Sedation was more common with haloperidol (13%) compared with placebo (3%). Insomnia also occurred more often with haloperidol (24%) vs. placebo (13%) indicating that the response can be unpredictable [45,48,49].

Loxapine

Most likely due to its high affinity for histamine H_1 receptors, loxapine is a relatively sedating, mid-potency first-generation agent. Sedation occurred at a rate of 32% with loxapine in studies comparing it with various other first-generation antipsychotics (i.e. chlorpromazine, perphenazine, and trifluoperazine,

Monitoring schedule for **SEDATION AND SLEEP DISTURBANCES**

Monitoring for sleep problems is to include direct questioning about insomnia (initial and maintenance), feelings of excess sleepiness during the day, and other sleep problems (e.g. restless legs, sleep walking).

	Baseline	Weeks		Months					Long-term monitoring
		1	2	1	2	3	6	12	
Second-generation antipsychotics									
Aripiprazole	•		•	•	•		•		⊛
Clozapine	•	•	•	•	•	•	•	•	⊛
Olanzapine	•		•	•	•		•		⊛
Paliperidone	•		•	•	•		•		⊛
Quetiapine	•		•	•	•		•		⊛
Risperidone	•		•	•	•		•		⊛
Ziprasidone	•	•	•	•	•		•		⊛
First-generation antipsychotics									
Chlorpromazine	•	•	•	•	•		•		⊛
Flupenthixol	•		•	•	•		•		⊛
Fluphenazine	•		•	•	•		•		⊛
Haloperidol	•		•	•	•		•		⊛
Loxapine	•	•	•	•	•		•		⊛
Methotrimeprazine	•	•	•	•	•		•		⊛
Molindone	•		•	•	•		•		⊛
Pericyazine	•		•	•	•		•		⊛
Perphenazine	•		•	•	•		•		⊛
Pimozide	•		•	•	•		•		⊛
Pipotiazine palmitate	•		•	•	•		•		⊛
Thioridazine	•	•	•	•	•		•		⊛
Thiothixene	•		•	•	•		•		⊛
Trifluoperazine	•		•	•	•		•		⊛
Zuclopenthixol	•		•	•	•		•		⊛

• Monitor for adverse effect. ⊛ As clinically indicated.

21%). Insomnia was less frequent with loxapine (3%) vs. risperidone (14%) in two studies [50].

Molindone

Molindone has a unique receptor-binding profile. It has relatively low potency for most receptors, which corresponds to its low rate of weight gain and extrapyramidal effects. Its receptor affinities also imply a low rate of sedation, although this was not observed in a recent treatment of early-onset schizophrenia spectrum disorders (TEOSS) study. Rates of sedation were 40%, 31%, and 32% with molindone, olanzapine, and risperidone, respectively. Among comparisons in small trials with other first-generation agents (i.e. chlorpromazine, haloperidol, and trifluoperazine), sedation occurred less frequently with molindone (25% vs. 37%) [51,52].

Perphenazine

Another clinically mid-potency agent is perphenazine. In the CATIE trial, it was associated with an intermediate rate of insomnia (25%) compared with ziprasidone (30%), risperidone (24%), quetiapine (18%), and olanzapine (16%). It was similarly intermediate in the rate of hypersomnia (sleepiness) (28%) compared with olanzapine (31%), quetiapine (31%), risperidone (28%), and ziprasidone (24%) [10].

Monitoring

Related to wakefulness, arousal, and sleep problems, the following should be assessed at baseline and monitored during treatment in patients taking antipsychotics:
- Insomnia: initial, middle, and number of awakenings
- Daytime sedation
- Naps
- Other sleep problems:
  - Restless legs
  - Periodic limb movements
  - Somnambulism
  - Night-time snacking/gorging

REFERENCES

1. Benson KL. Sleep in schizophrenia: impairments, correlates, and treatment. *Psychiatr Clin North Am* 2006;**29**(4):1033–45; abstract ix–x.
2. Krystal AD, Goforth HW, Roth T. Effects of antipsychotic medications on sleep in schizophrenia. *Int Clin Psychopharmacol* 200; **23**(3):150–60.
3. Silber MH, Ancoli-Israel S, Bonnet MH, et al. The visual scoring of sleep in adults. *J Clin Sleep Med* 2007;**3**(2):121–31.
4. Monti JM, Monti D. Sleep in schizophrenia patients and the effects of antipsychotic drugs. *Sleep Med Rev* 2004;**8**(2):133–48.
5. Tandon R, Shipley JE, Taylor S, et al. Electroencephalographic sleep abnormalities in schizophrenia. Relationship to positive/negative symptoms and prior neuroleptic treatment. *Arch Gen Psychiatry* 1992;**49**(3):185–94.
6. Goder R, Fritzer G, Gottwald B, et al. Effects of olanzapine on slow wave sleep, sleep spindles and sleep-related memory consolidation in schizophrenia. *Pharmacopsychiatry* 2008;**41**(3):92–9.
7. Miller DD. Atypical antipsychotics: sleep, sedation, and efficacy. *Prim Care Companion J Clin Psychiatry* 2004;**6** Suppl. 2:3–7.
8. Lu B, Budhiraja R, Parthasarathy S. Sedating medications and undiagnosed obstructive sleep apnea: physician determinants and patient consequences. *J Clin Sleep Med* 2005;**1**(4):367–71.
9. Seale C, Chaplin R, Lelliott P, Quirk A. Antipsychotic medication, sedation and mental clouding: an observational study of psychiatric consultations. *Soc Sci Med* 2007;**65**(4):698–711.
10. Lieberman JA, Stroup TS, McEvoy JP, et al. Effectiveness of antipsychotic drugs in patients with chronic schizophrenia. *N Engl J Med* 2005;**353**(12):1209–23.
11. Stahl SM. Antipsychotic agents. In Stahl SM, ed., *Stahl's Essential Psychopharmacology: Neuroscientific Basis and Practical Applications*, 3rd edn. New York, NY: Cambridge University Press; 2008.
12. Baldessarini RJ, Tarazi FI. Pharmacotherapy of psychosis and mania. In Brunton LL, Lazo JS, Parker K, eds., *Goodman & Gilman's The Pharmacological Basis of Therapeutics*, 11th edn. New York: McGraw-Hill; 2006.
13. Richelson E, Souder T. Binding of antipsychotic drugs to human brain receptors focus on newer generation compounds. *Life Sci* 2000;**68**(1):29–39.

14. Richelson E. Pharmacology of neuroleptics in use in the United States. *J Clin Psychiatry* 1985;**46**(8):8–14.
15. Luthringer R, Staner L, Noel N, et al. A double-blind, placebo-controlled, randomized study evaluating the effect of paliperidone extended-release tablets on sleep architecture in patients with schizophrenia. *Int Clin Psychopharmacol* 2007;**22**(5):299–308.
16. Nussbaum A, Stroup TS. Paliperidone for schizophrenia. *Cochrane Database Syst Rev* 2008;(2):CD006369.
17. McQuade RD, Stock E, Marcus R, et al. A comparison of weight change during treatment with olanzapine or aripiprazole: results from a randomized, double-blind study. *J Clin Psychiatry* 2004;**65** Suppl. 18:47–56.
18. Kane JM, Osuntokun O, Kryzhanovskaya LA, et al. A 28-week, randomized, double-blind study of olanzapine versus aripiprazole in the treatment of schizophrenia. *J Clin Psychiatry* 2009;**70**(4):572–81.
19. Zimbroff D, Warrington L, Loebel A, Yang R, Siu C. Comparison of ziprasidone and aripiprazole in acutely ill patients with schizophrenia or schizoaffective disorder: a randomized, double-blind, 4-week study. *Int Clin Psychopharmacol* 2007;**22**(6):363–70.
20. Kasper S, Lerman MN, McQuade RD, et al. Efficacy and safety of aripiprazole vs. haloperidol for long-term maintenance treatment following acute relapse of schizophrenia. *Int J Neuropsychopharmacol* 2003;**6**(4):325–37.
21. Tuunainen A, Wahlbeck K, Gilbody SM. Newer atypical antipsychotic medication versus clozapine for schizophrenia. *Cochrane Database Syst Rev* 2000;(2):CD000966.
22. McEvoy JP, Lieberman JA, Stroup TS, et al. Effectiveness of clozapine versus olanzapine, quetiapine, and risperidone in patients with chronic schizophrenia who did not respond to prior atypical antipsychotic treatment. *Am J Psychiatry* 2006;**163**(4):600–10.
23. Desarkar P, Goyal N, Khess CR. Clozapine-induced cataplexy. *J Neuropsychiatry Clin Neurosci* 2007;**19**(1):87–8.
24. Blum A. Triad of hyperthermia, increased REM sleep, and cataplexy during clozapine treatment? *J Clin Psychiatry* 1990;**51**(6):259–60.
25. Chiles JA, Cohn S, McNaughton A. Dropping objects: possible mild cataplexy associated with clozapine. *J Nerv Ment Dis* 1990;**178**(10):663–4.
26. Duggal HS, Mendhekar DN. Clozapine-associated restless legs syndrome. *J Clin Psychopharmacol* 2007;**27**(1):89–90.
27. Khalid I, Rana L, Khalid TJ, Roehrs T. Refractory restless legs syndrome likely caused by olanzapine. *J Clin Sleep Med* 2009;**5**(1):68–9.
28. Kang SG, Lee HJ, Kim L. Restless legs syndrome and periodic limb movements during sleep probably associated with olanzapine. *J Psychopharmacol* 2009;**23**(5):597–601.
29. Chiu YH, Chen CH, Shen WW. Somnambulism secondary to olanzapine treatment in one patient with bipolar disorder. *Prog Neuropsychopharmacol Biol Psychiatry* 2008;**32**(2):581–2.
30. Paquet V, Strul J, Servais L, Pelc I, Fossion P. Sleep-related eating disorder induced by olanzapine. *J Clin Psychiatry* 2002;**63**(7):597.
31. Kolivakis TT, Margolese HC, Beauclair L, Chouinard G. Olanzapine-induced somnambulism. *Am J Psychiatry* 2001;**158**(7):1158.
32. Kraus T, Schuld A, Pollmacher T. Periodic leg movements in sleep and restless legs syndrome probably caused by olanzapine. *J Clin Psychopharmacol* 1999;**19**(5):478–9.
33. Canuso CM, Dirks B, Carothers J, et al. Randomized, double-blind, placebo-controlled study of paliperidone extended-release and quetiapine in inpatients with recently exacerbated schizophrenia. *Am J Psychiatry* 2009;**166**(6):691–701.
34. Cohrs S, Rodenbeck A, Guan Z, et al. Sleep-promoting properties of quetiapine in healthy subjects. *Psychopharmacology (Berl)* 2004;**174**(3):421–9.
35. Calabrese JR, Keck PE, Jr, Macfadden W, et al. A randomized, double-blind, placebo-controlled trial of quetiapine in the treatment of bipolar I or II depression. *Am J Psychiatry* 2005;**162**(7):1351–60.
36. Srisurapanont M, Maneeton B, Maneeton N. Quetiapine for schizophrenia. *Cochrane Database Syst Rev* 2004;(2):CD000967.
37. Urbano MR, Ware JC. Restless legs syndrome caused by quetiapine successfully treated with ropinirole in 2 patients with bipolar disorder. *J Clin Psychopharmacol* 2008;**28**(6):704–5.
38. Pinninti NR, Mago R, Townsend J, Doghramji K. Periodic restless legs syndrome associated with quetiapine use: a case report. *J Clin Psychopharmacol* 2005;**25**(6):617–18.
39. Hafeez ZH, Kalinowski CM. Somnambulism induced by quetiapine: two case reports and a review of the literature. *CNS Spectr* 2007;**12**(12):910–12.
40. Zhong KX, Sweitzer DE, Hamer RM, Lieberman JA. Comparison of quetiapine and risperidone in the treatment of schizophrenia: a randomized, double-blind, flexible-dose, 8-week study. *J Clin Psychiatry* 2006;**67**(7):1093–103.
41. Wetter TC, Brunner J, Bronisch T. Restless legs syndrome probably induced by risperidone treatment. *Pharmacopsychiatry* 2002;**35**(3):109–11.
42. Lu ML, Shen WW. Sleep-related eating disorder induced by risperidone. *J Clin Psychiatry* 2004;**65**(2):273–4.

43. Prueter C, Luecke FG, Hoff P. Pavor nocturnus as a side effect of a single daily risperidone dose. *Gen Hosp Psychiatry* 2005;**27**(4):300–1.

44. Komossa K, Rummel-Kluge C, Hunger H, et al. Ziprasidone versus other atypical antipsychotics for schizophrenia. *Cochrane Database Syst Rev* 2009;(4):CD006627.

45. Leucht C, Kitzmantel M, Chua L, Kane J, Leucht S. Haloperidol versus chlorpromazine for schizophrenia. *Cochrane Database Syst Rev* 2008;(1):CD004278.

46. Essali A, Al-Haj Haasan N, Li C, Rathbone J. Clozapine versus typical neuroleptic medication for schizophrenia. *Cochrane Database Syst Rev* 2009;(1):CD000059.

47. Adams CE, Awad G, Rathbone J, Thornley B. Chlorpromazine versus placebo for schizophrenia. *Cochrane Database Syst Rev* 2007;(2):CD000284.

48. Hunter RH, Joy CB, Kennedy E, Gilbody SM, Song F. Risperidone versus typical antipsychotic medication for schizophrenia. *Cochrane Database Syst Rev* 2003;(2):CD000440.

49. Joy CB, Adams CE, Lawrie SM. Haloperidol versus placebo for schizophrenia. *Cochrane Database Syst Rev* 2006;(4):CD003082.

50. Chakrabarti A, Bagnall A, Chue P, et al. Loxapine for schizophrenia. *Cochrane Database Syst Rev* 2007;(4):CD001943.

51. Sikich L, Frazier JA, McClellan J, et al. Double-blind comparison of first- and second-generation antipsychotics in early-onset schizophrenia and schizo-affective disorder: findings from the treatment of early-onset schizophrenia spectrum disorders (TEOSS) study. *Am J Psychiatry* 2008;**165**(11):1420–31.

52. Bagnall A, Fenton M, Kleijnen J, Lewis R. Molindone for schizophrenia and severe mental illness. *Cochrane Database Syst Rev* 2007;(1):CD002083.

Seizures

Background

Schizophrenia is prevalent among people with epilepsy. Reported rates range between 4% and 18%, with the highest prevalence observed in people with temporal lobe seizures [1,2].

Most antipsychotics are associated with electroencephalographic (EEG) abnormalities, a lowering of the seizure threshold, and an increased risk of seizure induction at therapeutic doses. The most commonly reported seizure type with antipsychotics is generalized tonic–clonic. Myoclonic seizures without loss of consciousness or with subsequent progression to generalized tonic–clonic seizures are also linked to clozapine treatment [3–5].

Antipsychotic-induced seizures appear to be relatively uncommon in patients lacking risk factors. In patients not known to be at risk of seizures, the incidence of a first unprovoked seizure with antipsychotics is similar to that of the general population, estimated to be 0.073–0.086% [2].

Selected patient-related risk factors for seizure induction include epilepsy, brain trauma, brain mass, age, and electrolyte disturbance, especially hyponatremia. Drug-related risk factors include high antipsychotic daily dose, rapid upward titration of dose, and concomitant drug therapy with epileptogenic drugs. Drug–drug interactions resulting in higher serum levels of antipsychotics can also increase seizure risk [2].

Several methodologies have been used to determine the risk of antipsychotic-induced seizures, including EEG investigations, animal model investigations, and *in vitro* techniques using isolated brain tissue samples. The predictive value of these methods, however, is quite limited in general [2,6].

Agents of interest

Most first- and second-generation antipsychotics elicit dose-dependent seizure threshold lowering, indicating increased seizure risk at higher drug dosages and in overdose [2,7].

Antipsychotic agents have been found to induce EEG abnormalities resembling seizure activity at rates that far exceed the frequency of actual antipsychotic-induced seizures. These EEG abnormalities occur in the following order: clozapine (47.1%), olanzapine (38.5%), risperidone (28.0%), first-generation antipsychotics (14.5%), and quetiapine (0%) [4,8].

As a general rule, seizure risk varies with the sedative effect of the antipsychotic in that the more sedating the agent, the greater the risk of seizure. For an estimate of seizure risk derived collectively from clinical trials data, observational studies, and case reports refer to Table 1.14.1 [9,10].

Second-generation antipsychotic agents

Aripiprazole

The rate of seizures from short-term, placebo-controlled trials was 0.1% (3/2467) in adults and 0.3% (1/399) in youths (10–17 years). The rate with placebo was not available for comparison [13].

Table 1.14.1 Estimated seizure risk of antipsychotics [2–4,7,11,12]

High risk (>1.0%)	Intermediate risk (0.5–1.0%)	Low risk (<0.5%)
Chlorpromazine (≥1000 mg/day)	Chlorpromazine (<1000 mg/day)	Aripiprazole
		Fluphenazine
Clozapine (≥300 mg/day)	Clozapine (<300 mg/day)	Haloperidol
	Olanzapine	Molindone
	Quetiapine	Pimozide
	Thioridazine	Risperidone
		Trifluoperazine
		Ziprasidone

Aripiprazole has been implicated in causing seizures in two case reports [14,15].

Clozapine

Clozapine has the highest risk for inducing seizures among all antipsychotics. A retrospective study of patients treated with clozapine during the 16-year period prior to US Food and Drug Administration (FDA) approval (1972–1988) observed that 2.9% of patients had generalized tonic–clonic seizures. Seizure risk was found to relate to daily dose, with 1.0% at doses of <300 mg/day; 2.7% at doses of 300–599 mg/day; and 4.4% among patients taking ≥600 mg/day. Life-table analysis of these data predicted a 10% cumulative risk of seizure occurrence after 3.8 years of clozapine therapy [16].

A post-marketing 6-month study of the Clozaril® Patient Management System database reported a 1.3% incidence of generalized tonic–clonic seizures. Twenty-four of the 71 patients (34%) with seizures experienced recurrences. A dose–response relationship for seizures was reportedly not observed [5].

Severe myoclonus may precede and therefore warn of the onset of seizures with clozapine [17].

Olanzapine

There was a 0.9% incidence of seizures in premarketing trials of olanzapine. This ranks second to clozapine and slightly higher than other second-generation agents. Risk for seizures appears higher in people 65 years of age and older taking olanzapine [4,18,19].

Numerous case reports associating olanzapine with isolated seizures and status epilepticus have been published, but in many cases causation is difficult to determine due to the coexistence of various risk factors [4].

Paliperidone

Paliperidone is the active metabolite of risperidone. In short-term clinical trials, seizures occurred in 0.22% of subjects treated with paliperidone and in 0.25% of subjects treated with placebo [20].

Quetiapine

During premarketing trials, 0.8% of patients in the quetiapine treatment group developed seizures, while there was a 0.5% incidence in the placebo group and a 1% incidence in the active control group. The rate observed in clinical trials appears similar to that with olanzapine and higher than with aripiprazole, risperidone, and ziprasidone [2,19].

There are several case reports implicating quetiapine in the development of seizures [7].

Risperidone

Nine out of 2607 patients (~0.3%) developed seizures during premarketing trials of risperidone; two of the

Table 1.14.2 Putative drug- and patient-related risk factors for seizures [2,4]

Antipsychotic factors	Drugs associated with seizures	Patient factors
Sedating antipsychotic	Alcohol abuse or withdrawal	AIDS/HIV
Change in dosage	Amphetamines	Age (seizure incidence is higher in the
High maintenance dose	Antidepressants: bupropion, clomipramine,	geriatric population)
High serum drug levels	and maprotiline at therapeutic doses;	Central nervous system infections
High starting dose and/or	all tricyclic antidepressants (TCAs) in overdose	Cerebral arteriosclerosis
rapid dose escalation	Antiepileptic drug withdrawal (e.g. valproic	Hyponatremia or syndrome of
	acid, carbamazepine)	inappropriate secretion of
	Benzodiazepine or barbiturate withdrawal	antidiuretic hormone (SIADH)
	or rapid dosage reduction	Impaired drug elimination (i.e. reduced
	Carbapenems (e.g. imipenem)	renal or hepatic function)
	Cephalosporins	Organic brain damage or trauma
	Cocaine	Past or present electroconvulsive
	Isoniazid	therapy (ECT)
	Meperidine	Previous drug-induced seizure
	Penicillins	Previous personal or family
	Phencyclidine	history of epilepsy or seizures
	Theophylline	(including febrile seizures)
	Vaccines (febrile seizures)	

nine were associated with hyponatremia. The rate of seizures with risperidone appears to be the lowest among second-generation agents [19,21].

There are very few published case reports implicating risperidone in the development of seizures [7].

Ziprasidone

During clinical trials, seizures occurred in 0.4% of patients treated with ziprasidone, many of whom had contributing risk factors. The rate with placebo was not available for comparison. Relative to other second-generation agents, the risk of seizures with ziprasidone is low [19,22].

First-generation antipsychotic agents

Chlorpromazine and other phenothiazines

Of the first-generation antipsychotics, chlorpromazine appears to afford the greatest seizure risk.

In a 4.5-year observational study of hospitalized patients, 1.9% of 375 patients taking chlorpromazine

(median duration of use not stated) were found to experience at least one epileptic seizure. The overall rate with the use of all phenothiazines ($n = 402$, chlorpromazine, prochlorperazine, promazine, thioridazine, and trifluoperazine) was approximately 1.0% [12].

Seizure risk is dose related with chlorpromazine and presumably also with other phenothiazines. Seizures occurred in 0.3% of patients at doses of $\leq$200 mg/day of chlorpromazine or its equivalent, 0.7% at intermediate doses, and 9.0% among patients receiving $\geq$1000 mg/day of chlorpromazine or its equivalent. Seizures occurred most frequently in those with organic brain disease, shortly after initiating therapy, or following dosage increases (often within 2 weeks) [7,12].

Monitoring

Assessment of seizure risk factors, including concomitant drug use (prescription, non-prescription, natural health products, alcohol, and illicit substances) and

Monitoring schedule for **SEIZURES**

At baseline, assess risk factors for seizures. In follow-up, inquire about blackouts, observe for and inquire about myoclonus, and continue to assess risk factors.

	Baseline	Weeks		Months					Long-term monitoring
		1	2	1	2	3	6	12	
Second-generation antipsychotics									
Aripiprazole	•								⊛
Clozapine	•			•		•			⊛
Olanzapine	•								⊛
Paliperidone	•								⊛
Quetiapine	•								⊛
Risperidone	•								⊛
Ziprasidone	•								⊛
First-generation antipsychotics									
Chlorpromazine	•					•			⊛
Flupenthixol	•								⊛
Fluphenazine	•								⊛
Haloperidol	•								⊛
Loxapine	•								⊛
Methotrimeprazine	•								⊛
Molindone	•								⊛
Pericyazine	•								⊛
Perphenazine	•								⊛
Pimozide	•								⊛
Pipotiazine palmitate	•								⊛
Thioridazine	•								⊛
Thiothixene	•								⊛
Trifluoperazine	•								⊛
Zuclopenthixol	•								⊛

• Monitor for adverse effect. ⊛ As clinically indicated.

medical conditions, should be performed for all patients starting on antipsychotic therapy and repeated as clinically indicated. It is further recommended that seizure risk factors be reviewed for clozapine and chlorpromazine at 12 weeks.

For patients with multiple (two or more) risk factors (see Table 1.14.2), an antipsychotic with minimal seizure risk (Table 1.14.1) is preferred and should be started at a low dose and increased slowly to the minimum effective dose.

For all patients, the use of multiple high-risk agents should be avoided if at all possible.

For patients taking clozapine or moderate-to-high doses ($\geq$600 mg/day) of chlorpromazine, or for patients with one or more risk factors for seizures, it is recommended that regular inquiries be made regarding recent seizure activity early in the course of therapy or after substantial dosage increases.

When other drugs are added or removed, clinicians should consider the possible effect on the seizure threshold. For example, stopping drugs that increase the seizure threshold (e.g. valproic acid, benzodiazepines) can lead to seizures in patients with multiple risk factors who are taking an antipsychotic drug. Also, clinicians should be aware of drug–drug interactions that lead to an increase in the steady-state concentration of the antipsychotic. For example, adding an inhibitor (e.g. fluvoxamine and ciprofloxacin can reduce clozapine clearance) or stopping an inducer of the cytochrome P450 system (e.g. tobacco smoke induces CYP1A2) can result in an increase in the steady-state concentration of some antipsychotics. For an up-to-date list of potential cytochrome P450 drug interactions, refer to Dr. David Flockhart's list maintained by Indiana University's Division of Clinical Pharmacology at http://medicine.iupui.edu/flockhart/ [2].

Consultation with a neurologist is recommended when initiating antipsychotics in patients with a seizure disorder or a history of seizures. For this population, more intense monitoring for seizure activity is warranted when initiating an antipsychotic. Also, the possibility of drug–drug interaction between the antipsychotic and anticonvulsant needs to be assessed, as several anticonvulsants are known to induce or inhibit the clearance of antipsychotics. However, initiating an anticonvulsant prophylactically is generally not recommended in the absence of seizure history.

Identifying recent seizure activity

Suggestions for identifying recent seizure activity are:
Objective methods:
- Myoclonic jerks (myoclonic seizures)

Subjective methods:
- Have you lost consciousness recently (had a blackout or spell recently)?

REFERENCES

1. Gaitatzis A, Carroll K, Majeed A, W Sander J. The epidemiology of the comorbidity of epilepsy in the general population. *Epilepsia* 2004;**45**(12):1613–22.
2. Alldredge BK. Seizure risk associated with psychotropic drugs: clinical and pharmacokinetic considerations. *Neurology* 1999;**53**(5 Suppl. 2):S68–75.
3. Remick RA, Fine SH. Antipsychotic drugs and seizures. *J Clin Psychiatry* 1979;**40**(2):78–80.
4. Lee KC, Finley PR, Alldredge BK. Risk of seizures associated with psychotropic medications: emphasis on new drugs and new findings. *Expert Opin Drug Saf* 2003;**2**(3):233–47.
5. Devinsky O, Pacia SV. Seizures during clozapine therapy. *J Clin Psychiatry* 1994;**55** Suppl. B:153–6.
6. Yokota K, Tatebayashi H, Matsuo T, et al. The effects of neuroleptics on the GABA-induced Cl$^-$ current in rat dorsal root ganglion neurons: differences between some neuroleptics. *Br J Pharmacol* 2002;**135**(6):1547–55.
7. Hedges D, Jeppson K, Whitehead P. Antipsychotic medication and seizures: a review. *Drugs Today (Barc)* 2003;**39**(7):551–7.
8. Koch-Stoecker S. Antipsychotic drugs and epilepsy: indications and treatment guidelines. *Epilepsia* 2002;**43** Suppl. 2: 19–24.
9. Marks RC, Luchins DJ. Antipsychotic medications and seizures. *Psychiatr Med* 1991;**9**(1):37–52.
10. Herrmann N, Mamdani M, Lanctot KL. Atypical antipsychotics and risk of cerebrovascular accidents. *Am J Psychiatry* 2004;**161**(6):1113–15.
11. Pisani F, Oteri G, Costa C, Di Raimondo G, Di Perri R. Effects of psychotropic drugs on seizure threshold. *Drug Saf* 2002;**25**(2):91–110.

12. Logothetis J. Spontaneous epileptic seizures and electro-encephalographic changes in the course of phenothiazine therapy. *Neurology* 1967;**17**(9):869–77.

13. Bristol-Myers Squibb, Otsuka America Pharmaceutical. *Abilify (Aripiprazole) U.S. Full Prescribing Information.* Tokyo, Japan: Otsuka Pharmaceutical Co., Ltd.; 2008.

14. Malik AR, Ravasia S. Aripiprazole-induced seizure. *Can J Psychiatry* 2005;**50**(3):186.

15. Tsai JF. Aripiprazole-associated seizure. *J Clin Psychiatry* 2006;**67**(6):995–6.

16. Devinsky O, Honigfeld G, Patin J. Clozapine-related seizures. *Neurology* 1991;**41**(3):369–71.

17. Haddad PM, Sharma SG. Adverse effects of atypical antipsychotics: differential risk and clinical implications. *CNS Drugs* 2007;**21**(11):911–36.

18. Lilly. *Zyprexa (Olanzapine) Product Monograph.* Toronto, Canada: Lilly; 2008.

19. Alper K, Schwartz KA, Kolts RL, Khan A. Seizure incidence in psychopharmacological clinical trials: an analysis of Food and Drug Administration (FDA) summary basis of approval reports. *Biol Psychiatry* 2007;**62**(4):345–54.

20. Janssen-Ortho Inc. *Invega (Paliperidone) Canadian Product Monograph.* Toronto, Canada: Janssen-Ortho Inc.; 2009.

21. Janssen. *Risperdal (Risperidone) U.S. Full Prescribing Information.* Titusville, NJ: Ortho-McNeil-Janssen Pharmaceuticals, Inc.; 2006.

22. Pfizer Canada Inc. *Zeldox (Ziprasidone hydrochloride) Canadian Product Monograph.* Quebec, Canada: Pfizer Canada Inc.; 2007.

Sexual dysfunction

Background

According to the *Diagnostic and Statistical Manual of Mental Disorders*, 4th edn (DSM-IV), sexual dysfunction is defined as a disturbance in the sexual response cycle or pain associated with intercourse. The four components of the sexual response cycle are: (i) desire (fantasies, interest); (ii) excitement (erection in men, engorgement and lubrication in women); (iii) orgasm; and (iv) resolution [1].

Causes of sexual dysfunction can be psychological, pathophysiological, pharmacological, or multi-etiological. Determining and correcting the causes can be challenging to clinicians and is not always successful [2–4].

Sexual dysfunction is common in the general population. The 1992 US National Health and Social Life Survey found the rate to be slightly higher in women compared with men. In women, the primary problems were low desire, arousal problems, and pain. In men, the leading stated problem was premature ejaculation, with erectile dysfunction and low desire cited much less often [5,6].

The rate of sexual performance problems (37%) in untreated patients with recently diagnosed schizophrenia appears elevated compared with the general population [7].

A higher rate of sexual dysfunction appears to occur in older adults with schizophrenia being treated with antipsychotics. One community survey estimated the rate of at least one type of sexual dysfunction to be 82% in men and 96% in women with schizophrenia, compared with 38% and 58% of study controls. In this survey, prevalence of sexual dysfunction was not related to type of antipsychotic, i.e. first- or second-generation agent. Collectively, studies suggest sexual dysfunction rates in treated and untreated patients with schizophrenia to be 30–80% in women and 45–80% in men [2,8].

Prolactin elevation is a leading cause of sexual dysfunction associated with antipsychotics. However, prolactin changes do not explain all reported cases. Sexual dysfunction often exists in the absence of raised prolactin, suggesting that other mechanisms – biological and psychological – are involved. Prolactin-related adverse effects are detailed in Chapter 1.11 [2,3].

The pharmacological causes of sexual dysfunction in people taking antipsychotics are complex, multifaceted, and incompletely understood. Antipsychotics block several receptors related to sexual functioning. Dopaminergic activity is associated with sexual arousal; its blockade therefore may reduce desire and physiological response, directly and indirectly via prolactin elevation. Antihistamine effects can induce sedation and an associated loss of interest. Blockade of serotonin 5-HT$_2$ receptors in animal models has been shown to facilitate sexual behavior, while enhanced serotonin activity inhibits it. Antipsychotics with potent 5-HT$_2$ blocking effects (most second-generation agents) may therefore cause less sexual dysfunction than agents without this effect [2,3].

Several antipsychotics have been associated with priapism, a urological emergency. Onset is idiosyncratic, with no clear relationship to dose or duration of treatment. Although the risk is rare for this side effect with any agent, antipsychotics have been implicated in causing 20% of drug-induced priapism cases. Clitoral priapism is extremely rare, especially related to antipsychotics. Often patients report experiencing prolonged, painless erections before the onset of painful priapism. A history of priapism with other medications is the only clinically useful risk factor [2,9,10].

The proposed mechanism of priapism involves direct adrenergic α_1 receptor blockade and/or anticholinergic effects, both of which facilitate vasodilation and filling of the corpus cavernosa. Veno-occlusive, low-flow priapism leads to ischemia and potentially irreversible tissue damage and mechanical dysfunction [3,11].

Antipsychotics can also affect the activity of several hormones involved in reproduction, for example gonadotropin-releasing hormone (GnRH), luteinizing hormone (LH), testosterone, and estrogen. The primary underlying cause of this effect, although not necessarily the only cause, is drug-induced prolactin elevation [2,3,12].

Antipsychotic-induced sexual dysfunction is a major cause of poor quality of life, negative attitude towards treatment, and poor adherence. Despite this, sexual dysfunction is profoundly underestimated and infrequently addressed in practice. In one of the largest and longest naturalistic studies, the report of sexual dysfunction according to patient reports was 40%, whereas it was 3% based on physician assessment [2,13,14].

Agents of interest

The dearth of randomized trials systematically evaluating sexual function with follow-up of adequate duration limits the ability to make definitive statements regarding the relative risk of sexual dysfunction among antipsychotics. Findings from longitudinal, observational studies have not been consistent.

Second-generation antipsychotic agents

Aripiprazole

Aripiprazole is a partial agonist at dopamine D_2 receptors and is not associated with prolactin elevation.

Switches in treatment from prolactin-elevating antipsychotics leads to normalization of prolactin levels with aripiprazole, and can lead to a resolution of prolactin-related sexual side effects [2].

In one of the few randomized trials that systematically assessed sexual function, 555 patients were allocated to either aripiprazole or standard treatment, which was either olanzapine, quetiapine, or risperidone selected by the prescriber. Sexual dysfunction scores (measured by the five-item Arizona Sexual Experiences Scale) improved similarly with aripiprazole and quetiapine, and less so with olanzapine and risperidone. However, even for the group with the largest improvement (men taking aripiprazole), the clinical relevance of the 8.5% reduction in total score is questionable [15].

When adding aripiprazole to ongoing antipsychotic therapy or switching between agents, a clinically important improvement in sexual functioning was observed in a small ($n = 27$), non-comparative, open-label study. Sexual dysfunction improved for both sexes, but more so for men. Libido, erections, and orgasms all improved for men. Arousal, orgasm, and menstrual irregularities improved in women [16].

Markedly increased libido and sexual arousal has been reported with aripiprazole [17].

Aripiprazole has been linked with causing priapism in a few cases [10,18,19].

Clozapine

Considering the extensive clinical and research experience with clozapine, the scarcity of useful clinical reports assessing its effect on sexual functioning is surprising. Clozapine does not elevate prolactin and is expected to help resolve prolactin-related sexual side effects when switching between antipsychotics.

Despite its neutral effect on prolactin, sexual side effects including erectile and ejaculatory problems can occur and may be related to its potent α_1 adrenergic blocking and anticholinergic effects. One non-randomized, 12-week study showed a small reduction in sexual performance with clozapine that was not statistically different from that with olanzapine or risperidone. Another study found a similar level of sexual dysfunction in patients taking clozapine and haloperidol; however, the trial was too brief in duration and rates may have partially reflected sexual dysfunction associated with previous treatment [20,21].

Nearly a dozen cases of priapism have been published implicating clozapine therapy [10].

Olanzapine

In treatment-naive patients with schizophrenia, olanzapine was associated with more-favorable outcomes compared with risperidone and first-generation agents regarding libido and sexual function at 6 months of follow-up [7].

Switching patients with sexual dysfunction taking risperidone or first-generation antipsychotics to olanzapine can lead to improved sexual functioning [22].

Despite these advantages, the risk of sexual dysfunction remains high with olanzapine treatment, affecting up to half of those treated [14].

Olanzapine has been implicated in approximately 12 published cases of antipsychotic-induced priapism. It is the only second-generation agent to be linked to a case of clitoral priapism [10,23].

Paliperidone

There is little information about paliperidone's effect on sexual function. It is the active metabolite of risperidone and can be expected to cause similar but not more sexual dysfunction than risperidone.

Priapism has been reported with paliperidone use [24].

Quetiapine

Like clozapine, quetiapine has weak dopamine D_2 receptor binding affinity and does not affect prolactin. Prolactin levels usually normalize when treatment is switched from more potent D_2 blockers to quetiapine, which can help resolve prolactin-related sexual dysfunction.

Collectively, studies systematically assessing sexual dysfunction in patients taking quetiapine have found rates of 50–60%, which is lower than risperidone and first-generation agents and similar to those observed with olanzapine. However, the severity of dysfunction may be lower with quetiapine compared with olanzapine. The most common issue is reduced libido. Most studies are limited by their non-randomized, open-label, short-term follow-up designs [2].

A cross-sectional study of 238 patients with schizophrenia or schizoaffective disorder showed moderate to severe sexual dysfunction, as assessed by the Arizona Sexual Experiences Scale, in patients taking risperidone, quetiapine, and olanzapine. Scores were 19.7, 17.8, and 20.3, respectively. The difference favoring quetiapine over olanzapine had an effect size of 0.41 ($p = 0.04$), indicating a small to moderate clinical difference [25].

Priapism has been reported in five patients taking quetiapine [10].

Risperidone

The rate of sexual side effects is relatively high with risperidone compared with other second-generation antipsychotics and appears similar to the rates observed with first-generation agents, presumably due to its potent prolactin-elevating effect [2,7].

Risperidone broadly affects the sexual response cycle, including loss of libido, erectile dysfunction, ejaculatory difficulties, and impaired orgasm in men, and in women leads to amenorrhea, loss of libido, reduced lubrication, and impaired orgasm [2].

In an observational, 6-month follow-up study of treatment-naive patients, loss of libido was similar between risperidone (35.5%) and first-generation antipsychotics (38.7%) and higher than with olanzapine (17.8%). A similar pattern of antipsychotic-induced sexual dysfunction was also observed (17.6%, 16.7%, and 10.4%) [7].

In a 12-month follow-up observational study, the reported rates of sexual dysfunction were: haloperidol 71%, risperidone 68%, quetiapine 60%, and olanzapine 56%. Patients receiving risperidone were at least twice as likely to experience problems with sexual performance compared with quetiapine and olanzapine. Emergent menstrual disturbances including amenorrhea were higher with risperidone (28%) compared with olanzapine (15%) and quetiapine (13%). However, the high rate of loss to follow-up between 3 and 12 months of 18% with olanzapine, 30% with risperidone, and 42% with quetiapine calls into question the accuracy of these estimates [14].

Priapism associated with risperidone has been reported in approximately 20 cases, and may be due to risperidone's potent α_1 adrenergic blocking effect [10].

Ziprasidone

Data are lacking to characterize the comparative risk of sexual dysfunction with ziprasidone.

A 12-week, non-comparative trial prospectively assessed sexual function in patients with schizophrenia or schizoaffective disorder started on ziprasidone. Sexual functioning did not worsen in patients not previously treated with antipsychotics ($n = 15$). Sexual functioning improved in patients who switched from previous treatment (primarily risperidone and olanzapine) to ziprasidone ($n = 41$), 50% of whom were much or very much improved. After 3 months of treatment with ziprasidone, 20–30% of patients reported reduced libido, delayed or lack of orgasm, and erectile or lubrication problems, which was less than half the baseline rate observed in the treatment-switching group [26].

Ziprasidone has been implicated in a single case of causing spontaneous orgasms in a woman [27].

Ziprasidone has high affinity for blocking α_1 adrenergic receptors. Three cases of priapism have been published involving ziprasidone [10].

First-generation antipsychotic agents

Virtually all first-generation antipsychotics have been associated with sexual dysfunction including priapism [10,28].

In an observational study ($n = 213$), the rate of sexual dysfunction in patients taking first-generation antipsychotics (45%) was higher than general practice normal controls (17%) and lower than patients attending a sexual dysfunction clinic (61%). However, scores on the Sexual Functioning Questionnaire were similar between the first-generation antipsychotic group (mean 20.5) and the sexual dysfunction clinic group (21.5) and higher than the general practice group (12.6). Although differences among classes of agents tended to be small, some

trends were seen. In women, sulpiride had the greatest negative effect on libido and arousal. It also most adversely affected erectile function in men. The thioxanthenes (flupenthixol, zuclopenthixol) also caused more sexual dysfunction, especially when compared with haloperidol, which demonstrated the fewest problems overall. Arousal problems associated with aliphatic phenothiazines (chlorpromazine, thioridazine) were relatively low in women, but they caused the most impairment of libido in men. The results of this study need to be interpreted cautiously, as it was a non-randomized, non-blinded, single evaluation of sexual functioning [28].

Very rarely, first-generation antipsychotics (e.g. zuclopenthixol, trifluoperazine, and thiothixene) have caused spontaneous orgasms [27].

Chlorpromazine

Most reports of antipsychotic priapism involve chlorpromazine and thioridazine. However, the incidence is considered rare. Both have also been associated with retrograde ejaculation [3,10].

Haloperidol

In a 1-year, naturalistic, prospective study, the highest rate of sexual dysfunction was associated with haloperidol (71%) compared with risperidone, quetiapine, and olanzapine. Patients receiving haloperidol were two to four times more likely to experience sexual dysfunction, including loss of libido, impotence, and menstrual irregularities, compared with olanzapine [14].

Thioridazine

Like chlorpromazine, thioridazine is associated with priapism rarely, likely due to its potent α_1 adrenergic blocking effects, and can also cause retrograde ejaculation [3,10].

Other first-generation antipsychotics

Priapism has been reported with other first-generation antipsychotics, including but not limited to

Table 1.15.1 Changes in Sexual Functioning Questionnaire for Females (CSFQ-14-F) and Males (CSFQ-14-M) (with permission from [30])

Men	Women
1. Compared with the most enjoyable it has ever been, how enjoyable or pleasurable is your sex life right now?	1. Compared with the most enjoyable it has ever been, how enjoyable or pleasurable is your sex life right now?
2. How frequently do you engage in sexual activity (sexual intercourse, masturbation, etc.) now?	2. How frequently do you engage in sexual activity (sexual intercourse, masturbation, etc.) now?
3. How often do you desire to engage in sexual activity?	3. How often do you desire to engage in sexual activity?
4. How frequently do you engage in sexual thoughts (thinking about sex, sexual fantasies) now?	4. How frequently do you engage in sexual thoughts (thinking about sex, sexual fantasies) now?
5. Do you enjoy books, movies, music or artwork with sexual content?	5. Do you enjoy books, movies, music or artwork with sexual content?
6. How much pleasure or enjoyment do you get from thinking about and fantasizing about sex?	6. How much pleasure or enjoyment do you get from thinking about and fantasizing about sex?
7. How often do you have an erection related or unrelated to sexual activity?	7. How often do you become sexually aroused?
8. Do you get an erection easily?	8. Are you easily aroused?
9. Are you able to maintain an erection?	9. Do you have adequate vaginal lubrication during sexual activity (get wet)?
10. How often do you experience painful, prolonged erections?	10. How often do you become aroused and then lose interest?
11. How often do you have an ejaculation?	11. How often do you experience an orgasm?
12. Are you able to ejaculate when you want to?	12. Are you able to have an orgasm when you want to?
13. How much pleasure or enjoyment do you get from your orgasms?	13. How much pleasure or enjoyment do you get from your orgasms?
14. How often do you have painful orgasm?	14. How often do you have painful orgasm?

Scale: 5-point Likert: 1 – lowest frequency or enjoyment, 5 – highest frequency or enjoyment. For items 10 and 14, 1 – highest frequency, 5 – lowest frequency. Scoring on the three phases of sexual functioning: (1) Desire: items 2 + 3 + 4 + 5 + 6; (2) Arousal: items 7 + 8 + 9; (3) Orgasm/completion: items 11 + 12 + 13.

fluphenazine, perphenazine, haloperidol, mesoridazine, molindone, and thiothixene [10].

Monitoring

Systematic monitoring of sexual dysfunction in people taking antipsychotics is justified by its high prevalence in both sexes, effect on quality of life, negative effect on treatment attitude, and association with poor treatment adherence [29].

Several questionnaires are available to use clinically to support a structured assessment of sexual function and satisfaction. Two options are identified here:

- The 14-item Changes in Sexual Functioning Questionnaire (CSFQ-14: 14 items, <10 min, clinician administered) (see Table 1.15.1) [30]
- The Arizona Sexual Experiences Scale (ASEX: five items, 5 min, self-administered) [31]

The following components of sexual function should be regularly assessed in people taking antipsychotics:

Men	Women
Libido	Libido
Erection	Lubrication
Ejaculation	Orgasm
Satisfaction	Satisfaction
Pain	Pain
	Menstrual cycle

Monitoring schedule for **SEXUAL DYSFUNCTION**

Monitoring should include inquiring about erection and priapism risk in men, lubrication and menstrual cycle in women, and libido, orgasm, satisfaction, and pain in all.

	Baseline	Weeks		Months					Long-term monitoring
		1	2	1	2	3	6	12	
Second-generation antipsychotics									
Aripiprazole	•					•	•	•	⊛ ⑥
Clozapine	•			•		•	•	•	⊛ ⑥
Olanzapine	•					•	•	•	⊛ ⑥
Paliperidone	•			•		•	•	•	⊛ ⑥
Quetiapine	•					•	•	•	⊛ ⑥
Risperidone	•			•		•	•	•	⊛ ⑥
Ziprasidone	•					•	•	•	⊛ ⑥
First-generation antipsychotics									
Chlorpromazine	•					•	•	•	⊛ ⑥
Flupenthixol	•					•	•	•	⊛ ⑥
Fluphenazine	•					•	•	•	⊛ ⑥
Haloperidol	•					•	•	•	⊛ ⑥
Loxapine	•					•	•	•	⊛ ⑥
Methotrimeprazine	•					•	•	•	⊛ ⑥
Molindone	•					•	•	•	⊛ ⑥
Pericyazine	•					•	•	•	⊛ ⑥
Perphenazine	•					•	•	•	⊛ ⑥
Pimozide	•					•	•	•	⊛ ⑥
Pipotiazine palmitate	•					•	•	•	⊛ ⑥
Thioridazine	•					•	•	•	⊛ ⑥
Thiothixene	•					•	•	•	⊛ ⑥
Trifluoperazine	•					•	•	•	⊛ ⑥
Zuclopenthixol	•					•	•	•	⊛ ⑥

• Monitor for adverse effect. ⊛ As clinically indicated. ⑥ Every 6 months.

If prolactin elevation is suspected, obtain a morning fasting plasma prolactin level. For more information regarding prolactin elevation refer to Chapter 1.11.

Inquiries about erection duration should attempt to identify not only impotence but risk for priapism. Individuals who have experienced painful, prolonged priapism often have described recurrent, painless, long-lasting erections that began after starting antipsychotic treatment.

REFERENCES

1. American Psychiatric Association. *Diagnostic and Statistical Manual – text revision*, 4th edn. First MB, ed. Washington, DC: American Psychiatric Association; 2000.
2. Baggaley M. Sexual dysfunction in schizophrenia: focus on recent evidence. *Hum Psychopharmacol* 2008;**23**(3):201–9.
3. Baldwin DS, Mayers AG, Lambert A. Sexual dysfunction. In Haddad PM, Dursun S, Deakin B, eds., *Adverse Syndromes and Psychiatric Drugs*. Oxford, UK: Oxford University Press; 2004.
4. Aizenberg D, Modai I, Landa A, Gil-Ad I, Weizman A. Comparison of sexual dysfunction in male schizophrenic patients maintained on treatment with classical antipsychotics versus clozapine. *J Clin Psychiatry* 2001;**62**(7):541–4.
5. Laumann EO, Paik A, Rosen RC. Sexual dysfunction in the United States: prevalence and predictors. *JAMA* 1999;**281**(6):537–44.
6. Laumann EO. Erratum: Sexual dysfunction in the United States: revalence and predictors (*JAMA* [February 10, 1999] **281**(6):537–544]). *JAMA* 1999;**281**(13):1174.
7. Bitter I, Basson BR, Dossenbach MR. Antipsychotic treatment and sexual functioning in first-time neuroleptic-treated schizophrenic patients. *Int Clin Psychopharmacol* 2005;**20**(1):19–21.
8. Macdonald S, Halliday J, MacEwan T, et al. Nithsdale Schizophrenia Surveys 24: sexual dysfunction. Case–control study. *Br J Psychiatry* 2003;**182**:50–6.
9. Patel AG, Mukherji K, Lee A. Priapism associated with psychotropic drugs. *Br J Hosp Med* 1996;**55**(6):315–19.
10. Sood S, James W, Bailon MJ. Priapism associated with atypical antipsychotic medications: a review. *Int Clin Psychopharmacol* 2008;**23**(1):9–17.
11. Segraves RT. Effects of psychotropic drugs on human erection and ejaculation. *Arch Gen Psychiatry* 1989;**46**(3):275–84.
12. Konarzewska B, Wolczynski S, Szulc A, Galinska B, Poplawska R, Waszkiewicz N. Effect of risperidone and olanzapine on reproductive hormones, psychopathology and sexual functioning in male patients with schizophrenia. *Psychoneuroendocrinology* 2009;**34**(1):129–39.
13. Dossenbach M, Hodge A, Anders M, et al. Prevalence of sexual dysfunction in patients with schizophrenia: international variation and underestimation. *Int J Neuropsychopharmacol* 2005;**8**(2):195–201.
14. Dossenbach M, Dyachkova Y, Pirildar S, et al. Effects of atypical and typical antipsychotic treatments on sexual function in patients with schizophrenia: 12-month results from the Intercontinental Schizophrenia Outpatient Health Outcomes (IC-SOHO) study. *Eur Psychiatry* 2006;**21**(4):251–8.
15. Hanssens L, L'Italien G, Loze JY, Marcus RN, Pans M, Kerselaers W. The effect of antipsychotic medication on sexual function and serum prolactin levels in community-treated schizophrenic patients: results from the Schizophrenia Trial of Aripiprazole (STAR) study (NCT00237913). *BMC Psychiatry* 2008;**8**:95.
16. Mir A, Shivakumar K, Williamson RJ, McAllister V, O'Keane V, Aitchison KJ. Change in sexual dysfunction with aripiprazole: a switching or add-on study. *J Psychopharmacol* 2008;**22**(3):244–53.
17. Schlachetzki JC, Langosch JM. Aripiprazole induced hypersexuality in a 24-year-old female patient with schizoaffective disorder? *J Clin Psychopharmacol* 2008;**28**(5):567–8.
18. Mago R, Anolik R, Johnson RA, Kunkel EJ. Recurrent priapism associated with use of aripiprazole. *J Clin Psychiatry* 2006;**67**(9):1471–2.
19. Aguilar-Shea AL, Palomero-Juan I, Sierra Santos L, Gallardo-Mayo C. Aripiprazole and priapism. *Aten Primaria* 2009;**41**(4):230–1.
20. Strous RD, Kupchik M, Roitman S, et al. Comparison between risperidone, olanzapine, and clozapine in the management of chronic schizophrenia: a naturalistic prospective 12-week observational study. *Hum Psychopharmacol* 2006;**21**(4):235–43.
21. Hummer M, Kemmler G, Kurz M, Kurzthaler I, Oberbauer H, Fleischhacker WW. Sexual disturbances during clozapine and haloperidol treatment for schizophrenia. *Am J Psychiatry* 1999;**156**(4):631–3.
22. Kinon BJ, Ahl J, Liu-Seifert H, Maguire GA. Improvement in hyperprolactinemia and reproductive comorbidities in

patients with schizophrenia switched from conventional antipsychotics or risperidone to olanzapine. *Psycho neuroendocrinology* 2006;**31**(5):577–88.

23. Bucur M, Mahmood T. Olanzapine-induced clitoral priapism. *J Clin Psychopharmacol* 2004;**24**(5):572–3.

24. Janssen-Ortho Inc. *Invega (Paliperidone) Canadian Product Monograph*. Toronto, Canada: Janssen-Ortho Inc.; 2009.

25. Byerly MJ, Nakonezny PA, Bettcher BM, Carmody T, Fisher R, Rush AJ. Sexual dysfunction associated with second-generation antipsychotics in outpatients with schizophrenia or schizoaffective disorder: an empirical evaluation of olanzapine, risperidone, and quetiapine. *Schizophr Res* 2006;**86**(1–3):244–50.

26. Montejo AL, Rico-Villademoros F, Spanish Working Group for the Study of Psychotropic-Related Sexual Dysfunction. Changes in sexual function for outpatients with schizophrenia or other psychotic disorders treated with ziprasidone in clinical practice settings: a 3-month prospective, observational study. *J Clin Psychopharmacol* 2008;**28**(5):568–70.

27. Boora K, Chiappone K, Dubovsky S, Xu J. Ziprasidone-induced spontaneous orgasm. *J Psychopharmacol* 2009; doi:10.1177/0269881108100321.

28. Smith SM, O'Keane V, Murray R. Sexual dysfunction in patients taking conventional antipsychotic medication. *Br J Psychiatry* 2002;**181**:49–55.

29. Kelly DL, Conley RR. Evaluating sexual function in patients with treatment-resistant schizophrenia. *Schizophr Res* 2003;**63**(1–2):195–6.

30. Keller A, McGarvey EL, Clayton AH. Reliability and construct validity of the Changes in Sexual Functioning Questionnaire short-form (CSFQ-14). *J Sex Marital Ther* 2006;**32**(1):43–52.

31. McGahuey CA, Gelenberg AJ, Laukes CA, et al. The Arizona Sexual Experience Scale (ASEX): reliability and validity. *J Sex Marital Ther* 2000;**26**(1):25–40.

Sialorrhea

Background

Sialorrhea (drooling) is a socially embarrassing and poorly understood adverse effect that has been linked to selected first- and second-generation antipsychotic agents. Paradoxically, it occurs most frequently with clozapine, a highly anticholinergic agent [1].

The mechanism of hypersalivation with clozapine likely differs from that of other antipsychotics, especially high-potency D_2 dopamine blockers. Clozapine is an antagonist at muscarinic M_3 receptors, an agonist at muscarinic M_4 receptors, and an antagonist at adrenergic α_2 receptors. Its effects on M_4 and α_2 receptors have been proposed as the mechanism of hypersalivation; however, several studies have failed to correlate subjective complaints of hypersalivation with increased salivary flow. Moreover, flow rates between those taking clozapine and normal controls appear similar and a single-dose study in healthy volunteers found a decrease in salivary flow with clozapine and no change with haloperidol. An alternative hypothesis describes dysfunction of the swallowing reflex caused by clozapine [2–8].

Salivary flow is primarily under parasympathetic cholinergic control and to a lesser extent is affected by sympathetic adrenergic innervation. Salivary flow increases almost fivefold with parasympathetic stimulation. Although muscarinic M_3 receptors predominate in salivary tissues, M_1 and M_4 receptors may also play a role in salivary flow control. Increased salivation is reported to occur through direct agonistic effects on adrenergic α_1 and β_1 receptors and muscarinic M_3 and M_4 receptors or by antagonism of adrenergic α_2 receptors [4–6].

When drooling is observed with high-potency D_2 dopamine antagonists, drug-induced parkinsonism should be considered as a potential cause.

Particularly with clozapine, sialorrhea often develops early and persists with chronic treatment. Drooling tends to be most severe during sleep. Patients will often complain of a wet pillow upon awakening, in addition to excessive drooling, choking, or gagging during sleep. Potential complications include sleep disturbance; irritated, macerated, or infected skin of the chin and perioral region; and, of most concern, aspiration pneumonia [2,9,10].

A variety of medical conditions (e.g. mental retardation, cerebral palsy, Parkinson's disease) and various drugs other than antipsychotics (e.g. cholinesterase inhibitors, bethanechol, lithium) are also associated with sialorrhea (Table 1.16.1) [1,11].

Agents of interest

Differences in research methodologies (e.g. different patient populations, length of studies, dosages used, methods of measuring salivary flow) and an absence of well-designed comparative studies prevent an accurate quantitative comparison of sialorrhea rates among different antipsychotic agents.

Despite the lack of evidence examining the link between sialorrhea and antipsychotics and the difficulty in estimating the incidence, the agents that appear to afford the greatest risk of sialorrhea in randomized controlled trials are clozapine, risperidone, and haloperidol.

Table 1.16.1 Causes of sialorrhea [1,11]

Conditions	Drugs
Neuromuscular/sensory dysfunction	Cholinergic drugs
Bulbar palsy	Bethanechol
Cerebral palsy	Cholinesterase inhibitors
Extrapyramidal syndrome	(donepezil, galantamine,
Mental retardation	rivastigmine)
Parkinson's disease	Antipsychotic agents
Stroke	Clozapine
Hypersecretory disorders	Haloperidol
Gastroesophageal reflux	Risperidone
disease	Other psychotropics
Idiopathic paroxysmal	Lithium
sialorrhea	
Oral inflammation	
(teething, dental caries,	
oral-cavity infection,	
herpes simplex virus 1,	
varicella-zoster	
virus)	
Anatomic	
Dental malocclusion	
Enlarged tongue	
Ill-fitting dentures	
Oral incompetence	
Orthodontic problems	
Other	
Foreign esophageal body	
Indwelling esophageal	
tubes	
Malignancy	

Second-generation antipsychotic agents

Aripiprazole

According to prescribing information, salivary hypersecretion occurred in 4% of adult patients treated with aripiprazole (15 mg/day or 30 mg/day) as an adjunct for bipolar disorder, compared with 2% receiving placebo [12].

In a pooled analysis of trials with pediatric patients (age 10–17 years) with schizophrenia or bipolar mania, salivary hypersecretion was reported in 4% of patients taking aripiprazole compared with 1% of patients taking placebo [12].

Salivary hypersecretion appears to be dose related. In a short-term trial involving pediatric patients (age 10–17 years) with bipolar mania, salivary hypersecretion was reported in 8.1% of the aripiprazole 30 mg group and 3.1% of the 10 mg group compared with 0% of the placebo group [12].

Hypersalivation and drooling was reported in a 27-year-old man with bipolar disorder with onset 3 months after starting aripiprazole. He was also taking sodium valproate. Sialorrhea resolved shortly after instituting trihexyphenidyl [13].

Clozapine

Sialorrhea is a very common side effect associated with clozapine, reported in 23–50% of patients. Patients describe drooling, a feeling of excess salivation, and choking. The odds of experiencing this side effect with clozapine are 6 to 12 times higher than with other antipsychotics [14,15].

Sialorrhea with clozapine is generally felt to be dose related, although not all studies have found a strong correlation. One small randomized controlled trial of 39 patients found an apparent dose relationship with the incidence of sialorrhea (0% at 100 mg/day, 32% at 300 mg/day, 48% at 600 mg/day). In another study, among nine patients taking 50–400 mg/day, there was no significant correlation between saliva flow rate and dose [2,4,16].

The exact mechanism of hypersalivation with clozapine remains unclear. Proposals of parasympathetic or sympathetic innervation stimulation, involving muscarinic M_4 agonist action and adrenergic α_2 antagonism have not been supported by saliva flow studies. An alternative and prevailing hypothesis is that clozapine interferes with normal deglutition, possibly by blocking target receptors in the pharynx or on the muscles involved in the swallowing reflex. However, this proposal remains theoretical as it is supported only by anecdotal findings of dysfunctions in swallowing peristalsis, sensations of nocturnal choking, and cases of aspiration pneumonia [2–4].

A possible complication of clozapine's hypersalivation is aspiration pneumonia. Cases of transient salivary gland swelling and parotitis have also been reported [9].

Olanzapine

Olanzapine appears to be associated less often with sialorrhea than the high-potency agent haloperidol (8.7% vs. 19.5%) (relative risk [RR] = 0.48; 95% confidence interval [CI] 0.39–0.59) [17].

In a randomized controlled trial ($n = 180$) comparing olanzapine and clozapine, the rates of hypersalivation were 2% and 29%, respectively [18].

Olanzapine has less of a risk of inducing sialorrhea than risperidone. In a large randomized controlled trial comparing olanzapine with risperidone, sialorrhea developed in 16.3% of patients taking risperidone compared with 6.4% of patients taking olanzapine ($p = 0.022$) [19].

Paliperidone

In short-term, fixed-dose, placebo-controlled trials, salivary hypersecretion is reported as occurring in 0% of patients taking 3 mg/day of paliperidone, <1% of patients taking 6 mg/day, 1% of patients taking 9 mg/day, and 4% of patients taking 12 mg/day compared with <1% of patients taking placebo. These data suggest that sialorrhea is dose related with paliperidone [20].

Paliperidone is the active metabolite of risperidone. Therefore, the risk for sialorrhea may be similar to that of risperidone.

Quetiapine

Other than two case reports, there is little information regarding hypersalivation with quetiapine [21,22].

Risperidone

In a randomized controlled trial comparing risperidone with flexible doses of haloperidol (mean dose 5.6 mg/day), there was no significant difference in the risk of hypersalivation (2.0% for risperidone vs. 4.8% for haloperidol, RR = 0.42, 95% CI 0.08–2.26) [18].

Risperidone is more often associated with hypersalivation than olanzapine (16.3% vs. 6.4%, $p = 0.022$) but less than clozapine (RR = 0.03, 95% CI 0.00–0.43) [18].

Ziprasidone

Increased salivation is listed as a dose-related adverse reaction in the prescribing information for ziprasidone. In short-term, placebo-controlled trials in patients with bipolar disorder, increased salivation occurred in 2.6% of ziprasidone-treated patients compared with 0.4% in the placebo group [23].

First-generation antipsychotic agents

Haloperidol

In two randomized controlled trials, the rate of sialorrhea was found to be significantly higher with haloperidol compared with olanzapine. In one trial, the comparative rates were 19.5% vs. 8.7% and in the other 6.2% vs. 1.2% [17,24].

Chlorpromazine

Sialorrhea does not appear to be a common problem with chlorpromazine, a low-potency, first-generation antipsychotic. In a 6-week randomized comparison with clozapine, 1 out of 142 patients (0.7%) taking chlorpromazine (≤1800 mg/day) reported sialorrhea when asked [25].

Monitoring

Before initiating an antipsychotic agent with significant potential for inducing sialorrhea (e.g. clozapine, haloperidol, risperidone), it is important to complete a baseline evaluation for the presence of drooling, a feeling of excess salivation, or swallowing problems. If present, review possible etiologies (see Table 1.16.1).

Monitoring schedule for **ANTIPSYCHOTIC-INDUCED SIALORRHEA**

Monitoring includes assessment of pre-existing and new-onset sialorrhea as well as for pre-existing causes of sialorrhea (e.g. medical conditions and drug therapy).

	Baseline	Weeks		Months					Long-term monitoring
		1	2	1	2	3	6	12	
Second-generation antipsychotics									
Aripiprazole	•								⊛
Clozapine[a]	•	•	•	•	•	•	•	•	⊛
Olanzapine	•								⊛
Paliperidone	•			•					⊛
Quetiapine	•								⊛
Risperidone	•			•					⊛
Ziprasidone	•								⊛
First-generation antipsychotics									
Chlorpromazine	•								⊛
Flupenthixol	•								⊛
Fluphenazine	•								⊛
Haloperidol	•			•					⊛
Loxapine	•								⊛
Methotrimeprazine	•								⊛
Molindone	•								⊛
Pericyazine	•								⊛
Perphenazine	•								⊛
Pimozide	•								⊛
Pipotiazine palmitate	•								⊛
Thioridazine	•								⊛
Thiothixene	•								⊛
Trifluoperazine	•								⊛
Zuclopenthixol	•								⊛

• Monitor for adverse effect. ⊛ As clinically indicated. ③ Every 3 months.

[a] Frequently screen for and assess the severity of clozapine-associated sialorrhea in the first 6 months of treatment. Monitoring can be reduced to every 3 months if sialorrhea is not considered problematic early in the course of therapy. After 1 year, if sialorrhea is not present, monitoring can be as clinically indicated.

At each visit for clozapine and as clinically indicated for other sialorrhea-inducing antipsychotic agents (e.g. haloperidol, risperidone), an assessment of drooling should be conducted, including gathering information from caregivers, if appropriate.

Suggestions for how to monitor

Objective assessment:
- Evidence of overt drooling noted by caregivers or in clinical settings
- Wet spot on pillow or bed linen upon waking, or on clothing at any time

Subjective assessment:
- Do you ever wake to a wet pillow in the morning?
- Do you ever notice yourself drooling during the day?
- Do you ever cough, choke, or gag on your own saliva (or wake from sleep because of this)?
- Has anyone ever mentioned to you that you drool?
- Do you feel you have to consciously swallow saliva in order to prevent drooling?

REFERENCES

1. Hockstein NG, Samadi DS, Gendron K, Handler SD. Sialorrhea: a management challenge. *Am Fam Physician* 2004;**69**(11):2628–34.
2. Praharaj SK, Arora M, Gandotra S. Clozapine-induced sialorrhea: pathophysiology and management strategies. *Psychopharmacology (Berl)* 2006;**185**(3):265–73.
3. Sockalingam S, Shammi C, Remington G. Clozapine-induced hypersalivation: a review of treatment strategies. *Can J Psychiatry* 2007;**52**(6):377–84.
4. Rabinowitz T, Frankenburg FR, Centorrino F, Kando J. The effect of clozapine on saliva flow rate: a pilot study. *Biol Psychiatry* 1996;**40**(11):1132–4.
5. Ben-Aryeh H, Jungerman T, Szargel R, Klein E, Laufer D. Salivary flow-rate and composition in schizophrenic patients on clozapine: subjective reports and laboratory data. *Biol Psychiatry* 1996;**39**(11):946–9.
6. Pretorius JL, Phillips M, Langley RW, Szabadi E, Bradshaw CM. Comparison of clozapine and haloperidol on some autonomic and psychomotor functions, and on serum

prolactin concentration, in healthy subjects. *Br J Clin Pharmacol* 2001;**52**(3):322–6.
7. McCarthy RH, Terkelsen KG. Esophageal dysfunction in two patients after clozapine treatment. *J Clin Psychopharmacol* 1994;**14**(4):281–3.
8. Pearlman C. Clozapine, nocturnal sialorrhea, and choking. *J Clin Psychopharmacol* 1994;**14**(4):283.
9. Davydov L, Botts SR. Clozapine-induced hypersalivation. *Ann Pharmacother* 2000;**34**(5):662–5.
10. Safferman A, Lieberman JA, Kane JM, Szymanski S, Kinon B. Update on the clinical efficacy and side effects of clozapine. *Schizophr Bull* 1991;**17**(2):247–61.
11. Boyce HW, Bakheet MR. Sialorrhea: a review of a vexing, often unrecognized sign of oropharyngeal and esophageal disease. *J Clin Gastroenterol* 2005;**39**(2):89–97.
12. Bristol-Myers Squibb, Otsuka America Pharmaceutical. *Abilify (Aripiprazole) U.S. Full Prescribing Information*. Tokyo, Japan: Otsuka Pharmaceutical Co., Ltd.; 2008.
13. Praharaj SK, Jana AK, Sinha VK. Aripiprazole-induced sialorrhea. *Prog Neuropsychopharmacol Biol Psychiatry* 2009;**33**(2):384–5.
14. Tuunainen A, Wahlbeck K, Gilbody SM. Newer atypical antipsychotic medication versus clozapine for schizophrenia. *Cochrane Database Syst Rev* 2000;(2):CD000966.
15. Wahlbeck K, Cheine M, Essali MA. Clozapine versus typical neuroleptic medication for schizophrenia. *Cochrane Database Syst Rev* 2000;(2):CD000059.
16. de Leon J, Odom-White A, Josiassen RC, Diaz FJ, Cooper TB, Simpson GM. Serum antimuscarinic activity during clozapine treatment. *J Clin Psychopharmacol* 2003;**23**(4):336–41.
17. Tollefson GD, Beasley CM, Jr, Tran PV, et al. Olanzapine versus haloperidol in the treatment of schizophrenia and schizoaffective and schizophreniform disorders: results of an international collaborative trial. *Am J Psychiatry* 1997;**154**(4):457–65.
18. Bagnall AM, Jones L, Ginnelly L, et al. A systematic review of atypical antipsychotic drugs in schizophrenia. *Health Technol Assess* 2003;**7**(13):1–193.
19. Tran PV, Hamilton SH, Kuntz AJ, et al. Double-blind comparison of olanzapine versus risperidone in the treatment of schizophrenia and other psychotic disorders. *J Clin Psychopharmacol* 1997;**17**(5):407–18.
20. Janssen-Ortho Inc. *Invega (Paliperidone) Canadian Product Monograph*. Toronto, Canada: Janssen-Ortho Inc.; 2009.
21. Oulis P, Masdrakis VG, Karakatsanis NA, Kouzoupis AV, Papadimitriou GN. Quetiapine-induced dose-dependent

hypersalivation in mania. *Clin Neuropharmacol* 2009;**32**(1):56–7.

22. Allen S, Hoffer Z, Mathews M. Quetiapine-induced hypersalivation. *Prim Care Companion J Clin Psychiatry* 2007;**9**(3):233.

23. Pfizer Canada Inc. *Zeldox (Ziprasidone hydrochloride) Canadian Product Monograph*. Quebec, Canada: Pfizer Canada Inc.; 2007.

24. Beasley CM, Jr, Hamilton SH, Crawford AM, et al. Olanzapine versus haloperidol: acute phase results of the international double-blind olanzapine trial. *Eur Neuropsychopharmacol* 1997;**7**(2):125–37.

25. Kane J, Honigfeld G, Singer J, Meltzer H. Clozapine for the treatment-resistant schizophrenic. A double-blind comparison with chlorpromazine. *Arch Gen Psychiatry* 1988;**45**(9):789–96.

Skin and hypersensitivity reactions

Background

Adverse skin effects were recognized early with the introduction of chlorpromazine and continue to be of concern in treatment-related adverse effects with antipsychotics. The most frequent types of cutaneous reaction are exanthematous eruptions, photosensitivity, and skin pigmentation. These, along with pruritis and urticaria, can occur with any antipsychotic. Antipsychotics account for approximately 20% of all adverse cutaneous skin reactions caused by psychotropics. Refer to Table 1.17.1 for types of skin reactions associated with antipsychotics [1,2].

Severe and life-threatening hypersensitivity reactions with or without skin manifestations (e.g. erythema multiforme, Stevens–Johnson syndrome, drug hypersensitivity syndrome, drug hypersensitivity vasculitis, and exfoliative dermatitis) appear to occur rarely or very rarely with antipsychotics. Of this group, exfoliative dermatitis is the most likely and has been seen with nearly all antipsychotics [1].

Photosensitivity reactions to ultraviolet sunlight occur in two forms: the more common phototoxic reactions and the rare photoallergic reactions. Phototoxic reactions are usually severe sunburns presenting with erythema, edema, hyperpigmentation, and desquamation. They are thought to result from the production of phototoxic products that are deposited in the skin, for example the promazinyl radical formed in the presence of chlorpromazine. Photoallergic reactions are rare cell-mediated hypersensitivity responses that typically onset within 1–2 weeks of starting treatment, or 1–3 days after sun exposure. In these reactions, ultraviolet radiation is absorbed and chemically transforms the drug in the skin to a potent allergen. They usually present as a pruritic eczematous eruption, but can also be vesicular, lichenoid, bullous, or urticarial. Systemic complications are unusual [1,3,4].

Only a small proportion of adverse cutaneous reactions to antipsychotics are severe or life-threatening. Clinical features indicative of a more serious drug reaction include fever, confluent erythema, facial edema and central facial involvement, blisters, lymphadenopathy, shortness of breath, hypotension and mucous membrane involvement [1].

Agents of interest

Second-generation antipsychotic agents

Aripiprazole

A case of photo-onycholysis (separation of the distal nail plate from the nail bed) associated with olanzapine and exacerbated by aripiprazole has been reported as has a case of acne caused by aripiprazole [5,6].

Clozapine

Although seen much less frequently than with phenothiazines, clozapine can cause severe sunburns to skin exposed to ultraviolet light [1,7].

Table 1.17.1 Adverse cutaneous reactions associated with antipsychotic drugs [1]

Common	Severe and life-threatening	Other general cutaneous reactions
Pruritis	Erythema multiforme	Acne
Exanthematous reactions	Stevens–Johnson syndrome	Psoriasis
Urticaria	Drug hypersensitivity syndrome/reaction	Seborrhea
Fixed drug eruptions	Drug hypersensitivity vasculitis	Hyperhydrosis
Photosensitivity	Exfoliative dermatitis	
Pigmentation		
Alopecia		

Clozapine has been implicated in causing rare but serious cases of systemic cutaneous hypersensitivity reactions. Serum sickness-like syndrome was diagnosed in one patient who developed a severe hypersensitivity syndrome, including the formation of urticarial plaques on elbows, knees, and buttocks, as well as fever, diaphoresis, myalgias and arthralgias, facial swelling, and markedly elevated antimyeloperoxidase antibodies. Several other cases with overlapping as well as distinct features indicate that clozapine can be a rare cause of such serious reactions. These other cases included clozapine-associated Sweet's syndrome (fever, leukocytosis, and erythematous plaques), angioneurotic edema, erythematous macular rashes associated with pericarditis, pericardial tamponade, pleural effusions, polyserositis, and allergic asthma [8–11].

Clozapine has also been associated with pruritis, urticaria, exanthematous reactions, erythema multiforme, and Stevens–Johnson syndrome [1].

Olanzapine

Case reports have implicated olanzapine in cases of photo-onycholysis affecting the fingernails, exanthematous pustular rash, and skin hyperpigmentation. In the latter case of acral melanosis, skin pigmentation in the affected 26-year-old man was described as slate gray and was limited in its distribution to the dorsal aspect of the hands [5,12,13].

Olanzapine has also been associated with pruritis, urticaria, other exanthematous reactions, fixed drug eruptions, other photosensitivity reactions, drug hypersensitivity reactions, alopecia, seborrhea, and hyperhydrosis [1].

Paliperidone

Paliperidone is the active metabolite of risperidone. It is possible that paliperidone causes the same adverse cutaneous reactions as risperidone.

Quetiapine

Quetiapine's use has been associated with pruritis, exanthematous reactions, fixed drug eruptions, photosensitivity, exfoliative dermatitis, pigmentation, acne, hyperhydrosis, psoriasis, and seborrhea [1].

Risperidone

Risperidone appears to cause rash at a higher rate than several other antipsychotics. Its use has been associated with pruritis, exanthematous reactions, urticarial eruptions characterized by pruritic edematous papules and plaques, fixed drug eruptions, photosensitivity reactions, hyperpigmentation, erythema multiforme, exfoliative dermatitis, alopecia, psoriasis, and hypohydrosis [1,14].

Ziprasidone

Ziprasidone use has been linked to exfoliative dermatitis, exanthematous reactions, urticaria, photosensitivity reactions, and alopecia. Cases of urticarial angioedema and erythema multiforme also exist [1,15,16].

First-generation antipsychotic agents

The risk for any type of adverse cutaneous reaction with first-generation agents is approximately 5%. Under *in vitro* conditions, most phenothiazines (e.g. chlorpromazine, fluphenazine, levomepromazine, perphenazine, thioridazine, trifluoperazine) and thioxanthenes (e.g. flupenthixol, thiothixene, zuclopenthixol) are strongly phototoxic indicating the risk for UVA-induced photosensitivity reactions [17–19].

Chlorpromazine

A blue–gray discoloration of the skin occurs in 1.5–2.0% of long-term users of chlorpromazine and other low-potency phenothiazines such as thioridazine. Sun-exposed areas are generally affected. The hyperpigmentation can initially appear as a brownish tan that evolves over time to a slate-like metallic blue [14,20].

Haloperidol

Adverse cutaneous reactions appear to occur less frequently with haloperidol compared with other first-generation agents. However, cases of hyperpigmentation, contact dermatitis, exanthematous reactions, fixed drug eruptions, phototoxicity, acne, and alopecia have been reported [1,14].

Loxapine

Loxapine use has been associated with pruritis, exanthematous reactions, seborrhea, and alopecia [1].

Perphenazine

See chlorpromazine and the general comments regarding first-generation agents.

Thioridazine

An antineutrophil cytoplasm antibodies (ANCA)-positive thioridazine-induced cutaneous leukocytoclastic vasculitis was observed in a 38-year-old man with schizophrenia [21]. For other possible reactions, see chlorpromazine and the general comments regarding first-generation agents.

Monitoring

≤1 month	Inquire about new-onset rash, itch, fever
General	Monitor for insidious-onset adverse effects (e.g. hyperpigmentation, alopecia, acne)
Sunny weather	Assess sun-exposed skin for indications of photosensitivity reactions (e.g. sunburn, hyperpigmentation)
Serious adverse cutaneous reactions	Inform patient of indicators of a potentially serious adverse skin effect: Fever Confluent erythema Facial edema and central facial involvement Blisters Lymphadenopathy Shortness of breath Hypotension Mucous membrane involvement

Monitoring schedule for **SKIN AND HYPERSENSITIVITY REACTIONS**

Monitoring for adverse cutaneous effects requires that the patient be aware of the possibility of rash and other immunological reactions. More insidious-onset skin effects, such as hyperpigmentation, acne, and alopecia, can be monitored for on a scheduled basis.

	Baseline	Weeks		Months					Long-term monitoring
		1	2	1	2	3	6	12	
Second-generation antipsychotics									
Aripiprazole	•			•			•		⊛
Clozapine[a]	•			•			•		⊛
Olanzapine	•			•			•		⊛
Paliperidone	•			•			•		⊛
Quetiapine	•			•			•		⊛
Risperidone	•			•			•		⊛
Ziprasidone	•			•			•		⊛
First-generation antipsychotics									
Chlorpromazine[a]	•			•			•		⊛
Flupenthixol[a]	•			•			•		⊛
Fluphenazine[a]	•			•			•		⊛
Haloperidol	•			•			•		⊛
Loxapine	•			•			•		⊛
Methotrimeprazine[a]	•			•			•		⊛
Molindone	•			•			•		⊛
Pericyazine[a]	•			•			•		⊛
Perphenazine[a]	•			•			•		⊛
Pimozide	•			•			•		⊛
Pipotiazine palmitate[a]	•			•			•		⊛
Thioridazine[a]	•			•			•		⊛
Thiothixene[a]	•			•			•		⊛
Trifluoperazine[a]	•			•			•		⊛
Zuclopenthixol[a]	•			•			•		⊛

• Monitor for adverse effects. ⊛ As clinically indicated.

[a] Monitoring for photosensitivity should be especially vigilant in spring and summer with the aim of prevention.

REFERENCES

1. Warnock JK, Morris DW. Adverse cutaneous reactions to antipsychotics. *Am J Clin Dermatol* 2002;**3**(9):629–36.
2. Lange-Asschenfeldt C, Grohmann R, Lange-Asschenfeldt B, Engel RR, Ruther E, Cordes J. Cutaneous adverse reactions to psychotropic drugs: data from a multicenter surveillance program. *J Clin Psychiatry* 2009;**70**(9):1258–65.
3. Harth Y, Rapoport M. Photosensitivity associated with antipsychotics, antidepressants and anxiolytics. *Drug Saf* 1996;**14**(4):252–9.
4. Kimyai-Asadi A, Harris JC, Nousari HC. Critical overview: adverse cutaneous reactions to psychotropic medications. *J Clin Psychiatry* 1999;**60**(10):714–25; quiz 726.
5. Gregoriou S, Karagiorga T, Stratigos A, Volonakis K, Kontochristopoulos G, Rigopoulos D. Photo-onycholysis caused by olanzapine and aripiprazole. *J Clin Psychopharmacol* 2008;**28**(2):219–20.
6. Mishra B, Praharaj SK, Prakash R, Sinha VK. Aripiprazole-induced acneiform eruption. *Gen Hosp Psychiatry* 2008;**30**(5):479–81.
7. Howanitz E, Pardo M, Losonczy M. Photosensitivity to clozapine. *J Clin Psychiatry* 1995;**56**(12):589.
8. Jaunkalns R, Shear NH, Sokoluk B, Gardner D, Claas F, Uetrecht JP. Antimyeloperoxidase antibodies and adverse reactions to clozapine. *Lancet* 1992;**339**(8809):1611–12.
9. Kleinen JM, Bouckaert F, Peuskens J. Clozapine-induced agranulocytosis and Sweet's syndrome in a 74-year-old female patient. A case study. *Tijdschr Psychiatr* 2008;**50**(2):119–23.
10. Mishra B, Sahoo S, Sarkar S, Akhtar S. Clozapine-induced angioneurotic edema. *Gen Hosp Psychiatry* 2007;**29**(1):78–80.
11. Bhatti MA, Zander J, Reeve E. Clozapine-induced pericarditis, pericardial tamponade, polyserositis, and rash. *J Clin Psychiatry* 2005;**66**(11):1490–1.
12. Christen S, Gueissaz F, Anex R, Zullino DF. Acute generalized exanthematous pustulosis induced by olanzapine. *Acta Medica (Hradec Kralove)* 2006;**49**(1):75–6.
13. Jhirwal OP, Parsad D, Basu D. Skin hyperpigmentation induced by olanzapine, a novel antipsychotic agent. *Int J Dermatol* 2004;**43**(10):778–9.
14. MacMorran WS, Krahn LE. Adverse cutaneous reactions to psychotropic drugs. *Psychosomatics* 1997;**38**(5):413–22.
15. Akkaya C, Sarandol A, Aydogan K, Kirli S. Urticaria and angio-oedema due to ziprasidone. *J Psychopharmacol* 2007;**21**(5):550–2.
16. Nobrega LPC, Baldacara L, Kumagai F, Freirias A, Tamai S, Sanches M. Drug eruptions associated with ziprasidone. *Rev Psiquiatr Clin* 2005;**32**(2):84–7.
17. Srebrnik A, Hes JP, Brenner S. Adverse cutaneous reactions to psychotropic drugs. *Acta Derm Venereol Suppl (Stockh)* 1991;**158**:1–12.
18. Chignell CF, Motten AG, Buettner GR. Photoinduced free radicals from chlorpromazine and related phenothiazines: relationship to phenothiazine-induced photosensitization. *Environ Health Perspect* 1985;**64**:103–10.
19. Eberlein-Konig B, Bindl A, Przybilla B. Phototoxic properties of neuroleptic drugs. *Dermatology* 1997;**194**(2):131–5.
20. Ban TA, Guy W, Wilson WH. Neuroleptic-induced skin pigmentation in chronic hospitalized schizophrenic patients. *Can J Psychiatry* 1985;**30**(6):406–8.
21. Greenfield JR, McGrath M, Kossard S, Charlesworth JA, Campbell LV. ANCA-positive vasculitis induced by thioridazine: confirmed by rechallenge. *Br J Dermatol* 2002;**147**(6):1265–7.

Tardive dyskinesia and other late-onset movement disorders

Background

Long-term use of antipsychotics can lead to delayed-onset movement disorders. Tardive dyskinesia (TD) is an involuntary movement disorder characterized by a variable mixture of dyskinetic movements typically involving the face, mouth, and tongue. Also common are tics, grimacing, truncal and axial muscle involvement, chorea, athetosis, and dystonias. Speech and respiration can be affected in severe cases. Also possible are tardive or chronic akathisia (a persistent sense of inner restlessness) and tardive dystonia (recurring, rapid-onset, often sustained muscle contractions causing abnormal twisting, contorting, and postures, e.g. torticollis, blepharospasm, oculogyric crisis, and spasms of the jaw, trunk, and extremities) [1,2].

Determining that these movement disorders are related to antipsychotic treatment can be challenging in the absence of a documented pre-treatment assessment, as a variety of neuro-medical conditions can present with similar features. It has also been observed that untreated patients with schizophrenia have a higher incidence of abnormal movement disorders [3].

However, the evidence implicating some antipsychotic agents as the primary cause of TD is beyond challenge. Most long-term studies of first-generation antipsychotics indicate that the rate of TD appears to be dependent on dosage and duration of treatment. Tardive dyskinesia can be irreversible. However, this risk is reduced when treatment is stopped or switched to an antipsychotic with low TD liability as soon as symptoms present [1].

Prevention and a rapid response to emerging signs of TD are vital in minimizing this side effect, as effective treatment modalities are lacking. Antipsychotics with higher liabilities for TD should be used cautiously or avoided in patients with risk factors. These include age (especially above the age of 50), female gender, the presence of affective disorders, development of parkinsonian side effects with antipsychotic treatment, high dosage, and prolonged treatment [1,4].

The mechanism underlying the development of TD and other late-onset movement disorders with antipsychotics most likely involves dopamine systems. The leading theory is dopamine receptor hypersensitivity. However, changes at the cellular and subcellular level are not well elucidated [5].

In an update from a 2004 systematic review, the annual incidence of TD with second-generation agents was estimated at 3.9% across all age groups (3.0% in adults). This is an increase from the previously reported 2.1% (0.8% in adults). The comparative rate with first-generation agents (primarily haloperidol) was reported at 5.5% [6,7].

The combined prevalence of severe forms of TD, tardive dystonia, and tardive akathisia with chronic, first-generation antipsychotic treatment is estimated at 1–5%. The combined risk with second-generation agents has not been reported. Methodological limitations of existing research prevent a more precise estimate [8].

Agents of interest

Differences in research methodologies (e.g. method of allocation, length of follow-up, dosage, measures and diagnostic criteria for TD) and significant variations in rates across different patient groups make it difficult to estimate TD risk accurately. There is a paucity of comparative studies with random treatment allocation available of sufficient duration to assess precisely the relative risk for TD among agents. The CATIE randomized controlled trial, which compared olanzapine ($n = 228$), perphenazine ($n = 229$), quetiapine ($n = 234$), risperidone ($n = 241$), and ziprasidone ($n = 134$) over 18 months, included the most comparators with a reasonably long follow-up. In patients with no evidence of TD at study entry, the annualized risk for new cases of TD (identified on two successive assessments) ranged between 0.7 and 2.2% among the second-generation agents and was 2.7% with perphenazine. The differences were not statistically significant [9].

Second-generation antipsychotic agents

At our Early Psychosis Program clinic, several patients (~2%) have developed tardive oculogyric crisis. Second-generation agents implicated include olanzapine, risperidone, and ziprasidone.

Aripiprazole

The rate of TD in premarketing clinical trials of aripiprazole was between 0.1 and 1.0% [10].

There are several reports of improvements or disappearance of TD with a switch to aripiprazole. There is also a case report of TD improving when aripiprazole was added to haloperidol [11–19].

However, there are also several cases of aripiprazole-induced TD [20–23].

Clozapine

Clozapine appears to have a very low liability for TD and other tardive movement disorders. Clozapine has been observed to reduce pre-existing TD with medication switches [24,25].

In an 18-week, randomized comparison of 90 people, no cases of TD were identified in patients with treatment-resistant schizophrenia taking clozapine, whereas ~2% developed TD while taking olanzapine [26].

Clozapine has also been reported to improve chronic akathisia [27].

Olanzapine

Among the five agents compared in the CATIE trial, at 1.1% olanzapine had the lowest observed rate of TD associated with it. The difference in rate was not statistically significant [9].

In a systematic review, the rate of TD with olanzapine ranged from 0% to 0.5% across two studies involving adults. In this review, no long-term data assessing the risk of TD in the elderly with olanzapine were identified [6].

The prevalence of TD has been examined in a 36-month, non-randomized, prospective study comparing olanzapine with risperidone, quetiapine, amisulpride, clozapine, oral first-generation agents, and depot first-generation agents. Drop-out rates were high and varied markedly across groups (from 33% with clozapine to 67% with quetiapine) bringing into question the accuracy of the findings. The prevalence of TD in the olanzapine group changed from 8.6% at baseline to 3.4% at the study endpoint, representing a 60% reduction. Reductions observed in the other groups were risperidone 39%, quetiapine 56%, amisulpride 51%, clozapine 42%, and depot first-generation antipsychotics 4%. The prevalence increased 6%, from 8% at baseline to 8.5% at endpoint, in the oral first-generation antipsychotic group [28].

In patients with pre-existing TD, switching to olanzapine has been associated with a significant reduction in TD over 8 months [29].

Paliperidone

Paliperidone is the active metabolite of risperidone. In the absence of long-term data, its risk for TD can be assumed to be similar to but not higher than that of risperidone.

Quetiapine

Among the five agents compared in the CATIE trial, at 4.5% quetiapine had the highest observed rate of TD associated with it when applying the Schooler–

Kane criteria of observing TD at two successive assessments. The difference in rate was not statistically significant [9].

In a systematic review, the 1-year estimated risk of TD with quetiapine was 0.7% in adults and 2.7% in the elderly [6].

In a 36-month, non-randomized, prospective follow-up study, the prevalence of TD was reduced from 12.1% at baseline to 5.3% at endpoint [28].

Risperidone

Among the five agents compared in the CATIE trial, at 2.2% the observed case rate with risperidone was intermediate [9].

A systematic review identified two studies that reported the annualized risk for TD with oral risperidone to be ≤0.6% in adults. For the long-acting injection of risperidone, a 1-year rate of 0.7% in adults was reported. In the elderly, the annual rate was estimated at 2.6% in one study (mean dose ~1 mg/day) and 13.4% in another (mean dose ~4 mg/day) [6].

A large, 36-month, prospective observational study reported either no change or a reduction, not an increase, in the prevalence of tardive movements from baseline to the finish across treatment groups. The rate dropped from 7.9% to 4.8% with risperidone [28].

Risperidone dose has been linked with the risk of TD in elderly patients [30].

Ziprasidone

Among the five agents compared in the CATIE trial, at 3.3% the observed case rate with ziprasidone was intermediate [9].

The annualized risk of TD with ziprasidone is estimated at 6.8% based on a single long-term study [6].

First-generation antipsychotic agents

Haloperidol

The risk for TD with haloperidol is particularly concerning. From a systematic review, the annual incidence of TD (mild to severe forms) with haloperidol was observed to be 5.4%. In another study, the 1-year incidence of probable or persistent TD in a cohort of first-episode psychosis patients treated with low-dose haloperidol (1.7 mg/day) was 12% [6,31].

Perphenazine

Among the five agents compared in the CATIE trial, at 3.3% the observed case rate with perphenazine was intermediate. Although not statistically different, its estimated annualized risk was highest at 2.7% [9].

Other first-generation antipsychotics

There are no data to suggest an important difference in TD risk among first-generation antipsychotics

Table 1.18.1 Summary of tardive-onset signs and symptoms to screen for and monitor [2,32]

Tardive dyskinesia	Tardive dystonia	Tardive akathisia
Abnormal dyskinetic movements involving:	Abnormal movements (sustained muscular contractions, twisting, repetitive movements, and abnormal postures) typically involving:	Frequent or constant:
Cheeks and lips		Inability to stay seated
Fingers, hands, and arms		Pacing
Jaw		Rocking
Toes, feet, legs		Shifting of weight while standing
Tongue	Jaw	Objective impression of restlessness
Trunk	Neck	Patients may declare that remaining
Other movements:	Swallowing muscles	still is unbearable or that they feel
Blinking	Tongue	like they are going to
Grimacing	Trunk	jump out of their skin
Sighing	Upper and lower extremities	
Swallowing		

Monitoring schedule for **TARDIVE DYSKINESIA AND OTHER LATE-ONSET MOVEMENT DISORDERS**

Monitoring includes assessment of pre-existing, new-onset, or changes in involuntary movement problems. Assess for late-onset movement disorders, for example using the ESRS (see Chapter 1.6). More frequent monitoring may be indicated for selected patients (e.g. elderly).

	Baseline	Weeks		Months					Long-term monitoring
		1	2	1	2	3	6	12	
Second-generation antipsychotics									
Aripiprazole	•						•	•	⋆ ⑥
Clozapine	•						•	•	⋆ ⑥
Olanzapine	•						•	•	⋆ ⑥
Paliperidone	•						•	•	⋆ ⑥
Quetiapine	•						•	•	⋆ ⑥
Risperidone	•						•	•	⋆ ⑥
Ziprasidone	•						•	•	⋆ ⑥
First-generation antipsychotics									
Chlorpromazine	•					•	•	•	⋆ ③
Flupenthixol	•					•	•	•	⋆ ③
Fluphenazine	•					•	•	•	⋆ ③
Haloperidol	•					•	•	•	⋆ ③
Loxapine	•					•	•	•	⋆ ③
Methotrimeprazine	•					•	•	•	⋆ ③
Molindone	•					•	•	•	⋆ ③
Pericyazine	•					•	•	•	⋆ ③
Perphenazine	•					•	•	•	⋆ ③
Pimozide	•					•	•	•	⋆ ③
Pipotiazine palmitate	•					•	•	•	⋆ ③
Thioridazine	•					•	•	•	⋆ ③
Thiothixene	•					•	•	•	⋆ ③
Trifluoperazine	•					•	•	•	⋆ ③
Zuclopenthixol	•					•	•	•	⋆ ③

• Monitor for adverse effect. ⋆ As clinically indicated. ③ Every 3 months. ⑥ Every 6 months.

when comparing equivalent doses and exposure times [4].

Monitoring

Before initiating any antipsychotic agent, it is critical that patients be examined for the presence of abnormal movements and it is essential that the findings, whether positive or negative, be documented.

The risk for TD is higher with first-generation agents compared with second-generation antipsychotics. Patients treated with first-generation agents long term should be formally assessed for the development of TD and other late-onset movement disorders (e.g. tardive dystonia and akathisia) more often than patients taking second-generation agents.

For patients with pre-existing TD who are switched to an antipsychotic with low TD liability, more frequent monitoring of TD signs and symptoms are recommended to determine whether or not the abnormal movements are resolving.

Monitoring tools

The Extrapyramidal Symptom Rating Scale (ESRS) is a comprehensive abnormal movement measurement tool and is recommended for monitoring tardive movement disorders including TD, tardive dystonia, and tardive akathisia.

The ESRS can be used as an aid to help remind clinicians what signs and symptoms to look for and document, or it can be used more rigorously by clinicians to document not only the presence or absence of abnormal movements but also their severity and rate of change over time.

A copy of this scale can be found in Chapter 1.6. A summary of signs and symptoms to screen for and monitor is given in Table 1.18.1.

REFERENCES

1. Kane JM. Tardive dyskinesia. In Young RR, Joseph AB, eds., *Movement Disorders in Neurology and Neuropsychiatry*, 3rd edn. Malden, MA: Blackwell Science, Inc.; 1999.

2. Tarsy D. Akathisia. In Young RR, Joseph AB, eds., *Movement Disorders in Neurology and Neuropsychiatry*, 3rd edn. Malden, MA: Blackwell Science, Inc.; 1999.

3. Owens DG, Johnstone EC, Frith CD. Spontaneous involuntary disorders of movement: their prevalence, severity, and distribution in chronic schizophrenics with and without treatment with neuroleptics. *Arch Gen Psychiatry* 1982; **39**(4):452–61.

4. American Psychiatric Association. *Tardive Dyskinesia: a Task Force Report of the American Psychiatric Association*. Washington, DC: American Psychiatric Association; 1992.

5. Jenner P, Marsden CD. Neuroleptic-induced tardive dyskinesia. *Acta Psychiatr Belg* 1987;**87**(5):566–98.

6. Correll CU, Leucht S, Kane JM. Lower risk for tardive dyskinesia associated with second-generation antipsychotics: a systematic review of 1-year studies. *Am J Psychiatry* 2004;**161**(3):414–25.

7. Correll CU, Schenk EM. Tardive dyskinesia and new antipsychotics. *Curr Opin Psychiatry* 2008;**21**(2):151–6.

8. Gardos G, Cole JO. Severe tardive dyskinesia. In Young RR, Joseph AB, eds., *Movement Disorders in Neurology and Neuropsychiatry*, 3rd edn. Malden, MA: Blackwell Science, Inc.; 1999.

9. Miller del D, Caroff SN, Davis SM, et al. Extrapyramidal side-effects of antipsychotics in a randomised trial. *Br J Psychiatry* 2008;**193**(4):279–88.

10. Bristol-Myers Squibb, Otsuka America Pharmaceutical. *Abilify (Aripiprazole) U.S. Full Prescribing Information*. Tokyo, Japan: Otsuka Pharmaceutical Co., Ltd.; 2008.

11. Anonymous. Aripiprazole improves neuroleptic-associated tardive dyskinesia, but it does not meliorate psychotic symptoms. *Prog Neuropsychopharmacol Biol Psychiatry* 2008;**32**(5):1342–3.

12. Caykoylu A, Ekinci O, Yilmaz E. Resolution of risperidone-induced tardive dyskinesia with a switch to aripiprazole monotherapy. *Prog Neuropsychopharmacol Biol Psychiatry* 2009;**33**(3):571–2.

13. Duggal HS. Aripiprazole-induced improvement in tardive dyskinesia. *Can J Psychiatry* 2003;**48**(11):771–2.

14. Grant MJ, Baldessarini RJ. Possible improvement of neuroleptic-associated tardive dyskinesia during treatment with aripiprazole. *Ann Pharmacother* 2005; **39**(11):1953.

15. Lykouras L, Rizos E, Gournellis R. Aripiprazole in the treatment of tardive dyskinesia induced by other atypical antipsychotics. *Prog Neuropsychopharmacol Biol Psychiatry* 2007;**31**(7):1535–6.

16. Rajarethinam R, Dziuba J, Manji S, Pizzuti A, Lachover L, Keshavan M. Use of aripiprazole in tardive dyskinesia: an open label study of six cases. *World J Biol Psychiatry* 2009;**10**:416–19.

17. Sharma A, Ramaswamy S, Dewan VK. Resolution of ziprasidone-related tardive dyskinesia with a switch to aripiprazole. *Prim Care Companion J Clin Psychiatry* 2005;**7**(1):36.

18. Witschy JK, Winter AS. Improvement in tardive dyskinesia with aripiprazole use. *Can J Psychiatry* 2005;**50**(3):188.

19. Kantrowitz JT, Srihari VH, Tek C. Resolution of tardive dyskinesia after addition of aripiprazole to haloperidol depot. *J Clin Psychopharmacol* 2007;**27**(5):525–6.

20. Abbasian C, Power P. A case of aripiprazole and tardive dyskinesia. *J Psychopharmacol* 2009;**23**(2):214–15.

21. Evcimen YA, Evcimen H, Holland J. Aripiprazole-induced tardive dyskinesia: the role of tamoxifen. *Am J Psychiatry* 2007;**164**(9):1436–7.

22. Wang LJ, Ree SC, Chen CK. Courses of aripiprazole-associated tardive dyskinesia: report of two cases. *Prog Neuropsychopharmacol Biol Psychiatry* 2009;**33**(4):743–4.

23. Lungu C, Aia PG, Shih LC, Esper CD, Factor SA, Tarsy D. Tardive dyskinesia due to aripiprazole: report of 2 cases. *J Clin Psychopharmacol* 2009;**29**(2):185–6.

24. Tamminga CA, Thaker GK, Moran M, Kakigi T, Gao XM. Clozapine in tardive dyskinesia: observations from human and animal model studies. *J Clin Psychiatry* 1994;**55** Suppl. B:102–6.

25. Jeste DV. Tardive dyskinesia rates with atypical antipsychotics in older adults. *J Clin Psychiatry* 2004;**65** Suppl. 9:21–4.

26. Tollefson GD, Birkett MA, Kiesler GM, Wood AJ, Lilly Resistant Schizophrenia Study Group. Double-blind comparison of olanzapine versus clozapine in schizophrenic patients clinically eligible for treatment with clozapine. *Biol Psychiatry* 2001;**49**(1):52–63.

27. Spivak B, Mester R, Abesgaus J, et al. Clozapine treatment for neuroleptic-induced tardive dyskinesia, parkinsonism, and chronic akathisia in schizophrenic patients. *J Clin Psychiatry* 1997;**58**(7):318–22.

28. Novick D, Haro JM, Perrin E, Suarez D, Texeira JM. Tolerability of outpatient antipsychotic treatment: 36-month results from the European Schizophrenia Outpatient Health Outcomes (SOHO) study. *Eur Neuropsychopharmacol* 2009;**19**(8):542–50.

29. Kinon B, Jeste DV, Stauffer V, et al. Olanzapine improves tardive dyskinesia in patients with schizophrenia (abstract). In *155th Annual Meeting of the American Psychiatric Association*, May 18–23, 2002; Philadelphia, PA.

30. Jeste DV, Okamoto A, Napolitano J, Kane JM, Martinez RA. Low incidence of persistent tardive dyskinesia in elderly patients with dementia treated with risperidone. *Am J Psychiatry* 2000;**157**(7):1150–5.

31. Oosthuizen PP, Emsley RA, Maritz JS, Turner JA, Keyter N. Incidence of tardive dyskinesia in first-episode psychosis patients treated with low-dose haloperidol. *J Clin Psychiatry* 2003;**64**(9):1075–80.

32. Adityanjee, Aderibigbe YA, Jampala VC, Mathews T. The current status of tardive dystonia. *Biol Psychiatry* 1999;**45**(6):715–30.

Urinary incontinence

Background

Urinary incontinence, or enuresis, is defined as an involuntary release of urine. Psychosis is a putative risk factor for urinary incontinence. It has been estimated that urinary incontinence occurs in 5–11% of hospitalized psychiatric patients [1,2].

Types of incontinence include urgency incontinence (a result of involuntary detrusor muscle contraction of the bladder), overflow incontinence (weak detrusor function or bladder outlet obstruction), and stress incontinence (insufficient bladder outlet resistance), which is the most common type and most likely the form associated with antipsychotic use [3].

Antipsychotics are associated with an increased risk of urinary incontinence independent of other risk factors. The rate of urinary incontinence in nursing home patients receiving primarily first-generation antipsychotic agents was found to be 1.7 (95% confidence interval [CI] 1.4–1.9) times higher than those not receiving antipsychotics [4].

Onset of urinary incontinence may occur within hours or days of the start of treatment or change in dosage, may diminish gradually without intervention, and can occur during the day or night. Urinary incontinence is often not reported by patients or detected by clinicians and is associated with non-adherence [1,5,6].

A history of childhood enuresis predicts a higher risk of antipsychotic-induced enuresis [2].

Multiple systems are involved in bladder control and voiding, including α and β adrenergic, nicotinic, muscarinic, serotonergic, and dopaminergic receptors,

among others. α_1-Adrenoceptors are located in the bladder neck and proximal urethra and when stimulated by norepinephrine cause an increase in bladder outlet resistance via an increase in smooth muscle contraction. Nicotinic receptors binding acetylcholine further increase outlet resistance; however, conscious, deliberate voiding activates parasympathetic muscarinic control, which leads to contraction of the detrusor muscle [3].

The mechanism of antipsychotic-induced urinary incontinence is not fully elucidated. It has been proposed that the combination of central dopamine receptor blockade and peripheral α-adrenergic receptor blockade causing urethral relaxation may contribute to the development of urinary incontinence. Studies of olanzapine and risperidone (in rats) suggest that several voiding parameters may be altered due to undetermined central pharmacological actions. It has been suggested that urinary incontinence associated with clozapine, especially transient cases, could be an indirect consequence of sedation [3,7–11].

Agents of interest

The incidence of antipsychotic-induced urinary incontinence is likely to be under reported in randomized controlled trials. Few prospective trials have been completed in which problems with urinary incontinence were directly assessed. Data mostly derive from case reports and small retrospective and prospective observational studies.

Second-generation antipsychotic agents

Aripiprazole

In three 10-week, placebo-controlled randomized controlled trials in elderly patients with psychosis associated with Alzheimer's disease, the rate of incontinence (primarily urinary incontinence) was reported at 5% with aripiprazole-treated patients compared with 1% in the placebo-treated group [12].

Clozapine

The rate of urinary incontinence of 1%, as reported by the product monograph, is lower than found by independent investigations and is likely to be a significant underestimation of this risk due to underreporting [7,13].

A retrospective study of 61 Chinese patients taking clozapine reported urinary incontinence in 44% of patients. Twenty-five percent experienced persistent incontinence, and 18% experienced daily and nightly episodes of incontinence [14].

A 12-month prospective study of 57 patients with schizophrenia or schizoaffective disorder found that 30% of patients treated with clozapine developed urinary incontinence. Risk was increased with the concurrent use of first-generation antipsychotics and in women [10].

A case report highlights the possibility of combined urinary and fecal incontinence. A 23-year-old man developed both urinary and fecal incontinence 2 weeks after starting treatment with clozapine. Symptoms stopped upon discontinuation of the clozapine and subsequently returned with rechallenge [15].

Olanzapine

In the CATIE trial (a large, double-blind, 18-month trial that randomized patients who were previously taking a variety of antipsychotics to treatment with olanzapine, risperidone, quetiapine, perphenazine, or ziprasidone), incontinence/nocturia was reported to have occurred in 5% of participants receiving olanzapine. The highest rate reported was 7% with risperidone and the lowest was 2% with perphenazine [16].

In a 6-week randomized controlled trial of 1996 participants with schizophrenia and related disorders, the relative risk of non-specific "urination difficulties" was 0.6 (95% CI 0.4–0.8) with olanzapine (13 mg/day) vs. haloperidol (12 mg/day), indicating a 40% reduced risk. The rates of "difficulties with micturition" were 4% and 6%, respectively [17].

A single case report describes urinary incontinence in a 61-year-old male with bipolar I disorder with psychotic symptoms associated with olanzapine therapy. Symptoms occurred after 4 days. Another describes urinary and fecal incontinence that developed within a few days of a dosage increase of olanzapine to 20 mg/day [18,19].

Paliperidone

There are no reports of urinary incontinence reported in clinical trials with paliperidone. However, given that paliperidone is the active metabolite of risperidone, its risk may be similar to but should not exceed that of risperidone [20].

Quetiapine

In the CATIE trial, incontinence/nocturia was reported in 4% of participants taking quetiapine [16].

Urinary incontinence was not reported as an adverse reaction in clinical trials completed by the manufacturer [21].

Quetiapine has lower affinity for α_1 adrenergic receptors than risperidone, clozapine, or olanzapine, and is a low-potency dopamine antagonist; as such, from a theoretical basis, it would be expected to cause less urinary incontinence than the other agents [3,22].

Risperidone

Undefined micturition disturbances were reported from clinical trials to occur in >10% of patients receiving risperidone [23].

In the CATIE trial, incontinence/nocturia was reported at a rate of 7% of participants receiving risperidone, which was the highest rate compared with perphenazine (2%), quetiapine (4%), olanzapine (5%), and ziprasidone (5%) [16].

In a 9-month observational study of 68 patients treated with risperidone, 28% reported urinary incontinence [24].

There are two case reports in pediatric patients who developed both urinary and fecal incontinence shortly after initiation of risperidone therapy, one within the first week and the other during the third week of treatment [25].

Data on the onset and course of urinary incontinence with risperidone are sparse. Based on case reports, onset can be as early as 1–4 weeks. There is little to indicate that this side effect is transient [6,25].

Relative to other antipsychotics, risperidone is a potent antagonist at α_1 adrenergic receptors, which may be the basis of its mechanism of urinary incontinence [3,22].

Ziprasidone

There were no reports of urinary incontinence during clinical trials involving ziprasidone [26].

In the CATIE trial, the rate of incontinence/nocturia in the ziprasidone-treated group was 5% [16].

First-generation antipsychotic agents

Chlorpromazine

Cases of urinary incontinence have been reported with chlorpromazine (300–800 mg/day) as monotherapy and combination therapy. Conversely, regimens of chlorpromazine 1200–1700 mg/day have been well tolerated by individuals who experienced urinary incontinence while receiving other antipsychotic medications [27,28].

Relative to other antipsychotics, chlorpromazine has a high affinity for α_1 adrenergic receptors, which may be the basis of its mechanism of urinary incontinence [3,22].

Flupenthixol

Flupenthixol-related urinary incontinence was demonstrated in a single case of a 35-year-old woman. Enuresis occurred within 7 days of receiving flupenthixol by depot injection, and then resolved with a prolonged interruption of treatment. Recurrent incontinence presented upon re-starting flupenthixol [29].

Fluphenazine

Three reports involving five adult patients have associated fluphenazine with urinary incontinence. Incontinence had occurred previously with haloperidol in one patient and in another was only a problem when fluphenazine was combined with chlorpromazine [27].

Haloperidol

Case reports describe urinary incontinence occurring in male ($n = 2$) and female ($n = 1$) adult patients within 4 hours to 3 days of receiving high doses of haloperidol (20–60 mg/day). Incontinence occurred within 4 hours in a patient who had received two 20 mg short-acting intramuscular injections [27].

Pimozide

A causal relationship with pimozide and enuresis was suggested in a 9-year-old boy treated with pimozide 3 mg at bedtime. Enuresis persisted for 1.5 years during pimozide therapy and resolved upon discontinuation [30].

Thioridazine

In a small case–control study of hospitalized psychiatric patients without dementia, urinary incontinence was associated with thioridazine ($p < 0.04$). Six out of 14 incontinent patients had received thioridazine compared with 2 out of 22 psychotic controls ($p < 0.04$) [2].

Two case reports of men aged 29 and 30 years describe nocturnal enuresis that presented within 24 hours to 1 week of treatment initiation with thioridazine 100–400 mg/day [31]. Another case report described a 49-year-old man who developed daytime incontinence and enuresis after initiation of treatment with thioridazine [32].

Reports of stress incontinence in women treated with thioridazine 500–600 mg/day with or without other antipsychotic agents exist [33].

Monitoring schedule for **ANTIPSYCHOTIC-INDUCED URINARY INCONTINENCE**

Monitoring includes assessment of pre-existing, new-onset, or changes in continence and risk factors for urinary incontinence.

	Baseline	Weeks		Months					Long-term monitoring
		1	2	1	2	3	6	12	
Second-generation antipsychotics									
Aripiprazole	•			•					⊛
Clozapine	•		•	•	•	•			⊛
Olanzapine	•			•					⊛
Paliperidone	•		•	•	•	•			⊛
Quetiapine	•			•					⊛
Risperidone	•		•	•	•	•			⊛
Ziprasidone	•			•					⊛
First-generation antipsychotics									
Chlorpromazine	•			•					⊛
Flupenthixol	•			•					⊛
Fluphenazine	•			•					⊛
Haloperidol	•			•					⊛
Loxapine	•			•					⊛
Methotrimeprazine	•			•					⊛
Molindone	•			•					⊛
Pericyazine	•			•					⊛
Perphenazine	•			•					⊛
Pimozide	•			•					⊛
Pipotiazine palmitate	•			•					⊛
Thioridazine	•			•					⊛
Thiothixene	•			•					⊛
Trifluoperazine	•			•					⊛
Zuclopenthixol	•			•					⊛

• Monitor for adverse effect. ⊛ As clinically indicated.

Other first-generation antipsychotics

Thiothixene and trifluoperazine have also been linked with urinary incontinence [5,31,34].

Monitoring

Data from clinical trials most likely far under report the rate of urinary incontinence with antipsychotics, and should not be considered as reliable.

Collectively, the available information suggests that urinary incontinence is infrequent with most antipsychotics but the risk appears higher with risperidone (and theoretically with paliperidone) and highest with clozapine, necessitating closer monitoring.

Although not associated with significant morbidity, urinary incontinence is associated with antipsychotic non-adherence. Due to the low rates of spontaneous reporting, clinicians should directly inquire about this adverse effect.

Questions to ask at follow-up include:

- "Do you have trouble with your bladder?"
- "Do you have trouble holding your urine (water)?"
- "Do you ever wake up having wet yourself?"
- "Do you have to change your under clothes?"
- "Do you ever wear a pad or other protection to collect urine?"

Antipsychotic-induced urinary incontinence may occur within days to weeks of treatment initiation or dosage increase. Clozapine-induced urinary incontinence may develop within 3 months of treatment. It is recommended that urinary abnormalities should be assessed at baseline and at 2 weeks for all agents. Risperidone-, paliperidone-, and clozapine-treated patients should be questioned for the first 3 months. Monitoring should continue as clinically indicated.

REFERENCES

1. Pollack MH, Reiter S, Hammerness P. Genitourinary and sexual adverse effects of psychotropic medication. *Int J Psychiatry Med* 1992;**22**(4):305–27.

2. Berrios GE. Temporary urinary incontinence in the acute psychiatric patient without delirium or dementia. *Br J Psychiatry* 1986;**149**:224–7.

3. Tsakiris P, Oelke M, Michel MC. Drug-induced urinary incontinence. *Drugs Aging* 2008;**25**(7):541–9.

4. Lindesay J, Matthews R, Jagger C. Factors associated with antipsychotic drug use in residential care: changes between 1990 and 1997. *Int J Geriatr Psychiatry* 2003;**18**(6):511–19.

5. Ambrosini PJ, Nurnberg HG. Enuresis and incontinence occurring with neuroleptics. *Am J Psychiatry* 1980;**137**(10):1278–9.

6. Agarwal V. Urinary incontinence with risperidone. *J Clin Psychiatry* 2000;**61**(3):219.

7. Lieberman JA. Maximizing clozapine therapy: managing side effects. *J Clin Psychiatry* 1998;**59** Suppl. 3:38–43.

8. English BA, Still DJ, Harper J, Saklad SR. Failure of tolterodine to treat clozapine-induced nocturnal enuresis. *Ann Pharmacother* 2001;**35**(7–8):867–9.

9. Vera PL, Miranda-Sousa A, Nadelhaft I. Effects of two atypical neuroleptics, olanzapine and risperidone, on the function of the urinary bladder and the external urethral sphincter in anesthetized rats. *BMC Pharmacol* 2001;**1**:4.

10. Fuller MA, Borovicka MC, Jaskiw GE, Simon MR, Kwon K, Konicki PE. Clozapine-induced urinary incontinence: incidence and treatment with ephedrine. *J Clin Psychiatry* 1996;**57**(11):514–18.

11. Warner JP, Harvey CA, Barnes TR. Clozapine and urinary incontinence. *Int Clin Psychopharmacol* 1994;**9**(3):207–9.

12. Bristol-Myers Squibb, Otsuka America Pharmaceutical. *Abilify (Aripiprazole) U.S. Full Prescribing Information.* Tokyo, Japan: Otsuka Pharmaceutical Co., Ltd.; 2008.

13. Novartis Pharmaceuticals Canada Inc. *Clozaril (Clozapine) Canadian Prescribing Information.* Dorval, QC: Novartis Pharmaceuticals Canada Inc.; 2007.

14. Lin CC, Bai YM, Chen JY, Lin CY, Lan TH. A retrospective study of clozapine and urinary incontinence in Chinese inpatients. *Acta Psychiatr Scand* 1999;**100**(2):158–61.

15. Mendhekar DN, Duggal HS. Clozapine-induced double incontinence. *Indian J Med Sci* 2007;**61**(12):665–6.

16. Lieberman JA, Stroup TS, McEvoy JP, et al. Effectiveness of antipsychotic drugs in patients with chronic schizophrenia. *N Engl J Med* 2005;**353**(12):1209–23.

17. Tollefson GD, Beasley CM, Jr, Tran PV, et al. Olanzapine versus haloperidol in the treatment of schizophrenia and schizoaffective and schizophreniform disorders: results of an international collaborative trial. *Am J Psychiatry* 1997;**154**(4):457–65.

18. Vernon LT, Fuller MA, Hattab H, Varnes KM. Olanzapine-induced urinary incontinence: treatment with ephedrine. *J Clin Psychiatry* 2000;**61**(8):601–2.

19. Sagar R, Varghese ST, Balhara YP. Olanzapine-induced double incontinence. *Indian J Med Sci* 2005;**59**(4):163–4.

20. Janssen-Ortho Inc. *Invega (Paliperidone) Canadian Product Monograph*. Toronto, Canada: Janssen-Ortho Inc.; 2009.

21. AstraZeneca Canada Inc. *Seroquel XR (Quetiapine fumarate) Canadian Product Monograph*. Mississauga, ON: AstraZeneca Canada Inc.; 2009.

22. Gardner DM, Baldessarini RJ, Waraich P. Modern antipsychotic drugs: a critical overview. *CMAJ* 2005;**172**(13):1703–11.

23. Janssen-Ortho Inc. *Risperdal (Risperidone) Product Monograph*. Toronto, Canada: Janssen-Ortho Inc.; 2008.

24. Vokas CS, Steele VM, Norris JI, Vernon LT, Brescan DW. Incidence of risperidone-induced incontinence [abstract]. *Schizophr Res* 1997;**24**(102):267.

25. Herguner S, Mukaddes NM. Risperidone-induced double incontinence. *Prog Neuropsychopharmacol Biol Psychiatry* 2008;**32**(4):1085–6.

26. Pfizer Canada Inc. *Zeldox (Ziprasidone hydrochloride) Canadian Product Monograph*. Quebec, Canada: Pfizer Canada Inc.; 2007.

27. Nurnberg HG, Ambrosini PJ. Urinary incontinence in patients receiving neuroleptics. *J Clin Psychiatry* 1979;**40**(6):271–4.

28. Alvi T, Reza H. Neuroleptic induced incontinence – case report. *J Pak Med Assoc* 1997;**47**(7):195–6.

29. Shaikh A. Urinary incontinence during treatment with depot phenothiazines. *Br Med J* 1978;**1**(6128):1698.

30. Shapiro AK. Pimozide-induced enuresis. *Am J Psychiatry* 1981;**138**(1):123–4.

31. Shenoy RS. Nocturnal enuresis caused by psychotropic drugs. *Am J Psychiatry* 1980;**137**(6):739–40.

32. Crittenden FM, Jr. Thioridazine incontinence. *JAMA* 1972;**219**(2):217.

33. Van Putten T, Malkin MD, Weiss MS. Phenothiazine-induced stress incontinence. *J Urol* 1973;**109**(4):625–6.

34. Kiruluta HG, Andrews K. Urinary incontinence secondary to drugs. *Urology* 1983;**22**(1):88–90.

Venous thromboembolism

Background

Venous thromboembolism (VTE) refers to two distinct conditions – deep-vein thrombosis (DVT) and pulmonary embolism. The annual incidence of VTE in the general population is estimated to be 0.1%. This rate increases from approximately 0.01% in young adults to 1% in the elderly [1].

Most cases of pulmonary embolism develop from proximal DVTs involving the popliteal, femoral, or iliac veins. Three factors are involved in the development of VTE: damage to vessel walls, venous stasis, and hypercoagulability, which are collectively referred to as Virchow's triad [1–5].

Mortality rates associated with VTE range considerably depending on the population studied and clot location. Generally, the rate ranges from 2.5% to 28% and may be higher in select groups (e.g. 78–90% mortality rate in patients with pulmonary embolism and cardiac arrest) [3,6].

Observational studies conducted in patients with schizophrenia suggest that this population is at increased risk of VTE compared with the general population. It is unknown whether schizophrenia itself confers a higher incidence of VTE or whether other factors, such as lifestyle or antipsychotic medications, contribute to the risk. For a list of risk factors for VTE, refer to Table 1.20.1 [7].

The incidence of VTE in patients with schizophrenia has not been measured precisely. Most studies of VTE are investigational autopsies and, as such, may not provide an accurate estimate of risk in patients with schizophrenia [7].

Several mechanisms by which antipsychotic agents lead to VTE have been postulated. Theories include sedation leading to immobility and venous stasis, obesity and associated reduced mobility, decreased fibrinolytic activity, anticardiolipin antibody production, and enhanced platelet aggregation [4,7–10].

In a hospital-based case–control study that included 677 cases and matched controls (mean age of both groups was 68 years), exposure to antipsychotic drugs was associated with more than a threefold increase in risk for VTE (odds ratio [OR] = 3.5, 95% confidence interval [CI] 2.0–6.2). There are also numerous case reports, several implicating newer antipsychotics, of VTE associated with antipsychotic use [11].

Agents of interest

Due to its apparent rarity and various degrees of severity and sequelae, an accurate estimate of the incidence of antipsychotic-associated VTE is unknown. As most data come from spontaneously reported cases, it is likely that the true incidence is underestimated by these reports. However, without reliable data, for example from large, prospective cohort studies, a true cause–effect relationship that demonstrates an increase in the rate of VTEs beyond the baseline risk in patients taking antipsychotics cannot be confirmed [7].

Second-generation antipsychotic agents

Several case reports, case series, and systematic studies describing the association between VTE and second-generation antipsychotic use are known [7,11,13].

Aripiprazole

Aripiprazole was not associated with VTEs during clinical trials and there have been no reports in the literature [14].

Clozapine

Numerous cases of clozapine-associated VTE have been published and reported to national registries in numerous countries including Australia, Canada, Germany, Sweden, Switzerland, and the USA [7,15,16].

Between 1990 and 1999, the US Food and Drug Administration (FDA) received 99 reports of VTE associated with clozapine use. The median duration of therapy prior to VTE was 3 months [17].

Twelve cases of venous thrombosis (six were pulmonary emboli) were spontaneously reported in Sweden between 1989 and 2000. This rate (at least 1 in 2000–6000) was estimated to be higher than that observed in patients taking other antipsychotics, although a causal association could not be established [15].

Olanzapine

Several cases of VTE associated with olanzapine have been reported, including a report of a 28-year-old man who developed a pulmonary embolism 10 weeks after initiating olanzapine [18].

In a case series, olanzapine was associated with pulmonary embolism development within 2 months of treatment initiation in three patients, aged 78, 84, and 89 [13].

Another case series describes four patients (aged 37, 53, 53, and 54) who had DVTs while on olanzapine. One of these patients went on to develop a pulmonary embolism [19].

A 25-year-old man with early-onset schizoaffective disorder developed pulmonary emboli on three separate occasions, the first 12 weeks after initiation of olanzapine and then twice while on risperidone [20].

Another case reported the development of a pulmonary embolism 3 months after a 28-year-old male was started on olanzapine (5 mg/day) for bipolar disorder [21].

A 54-year-old Japanese woman with schizoaffective disorder developed several DVTs and a pulmonary embolism 6 months after initiation of olanzapine therapy as augmentation for manic symptoms. She was also on several other medications including haloperidol, levomepromazine, and promethazine [22].

Paliperidone

Paliperidone was not associated with VTEs during premarketing evaluation. No cases were identified in the literature [23].

Paliperidone is the active metabolite of risperidone. Its risk for VTE may be similar to that of risperidone.

Table 1.20.1 Risk factors associated with VTE [2,12]

Acute medical illness	Drugs:
Advancing age (>40 years)	Cancer therapy
Central venous catheterization	Estrogen
	Selective estrogen receptor modulators
Heart or respiratory failure	Inherited or acquired thrombophilias:
History of prior thromboembolic event	Activated protein C resistance
Immobility or paralysis	Dysfibrinogenemia
Inflammatory bowel disease	Protein C, protein S, or antithrombin deficiency
Malignancy	Prothrombin G20210A
Myeloproliferative disorder	Recent:
	Myocardial infarction
Nephrotic syndrome	Surgery
Obesity	Trauma
Paroxysmal nocturnal hemoglobinuria	
Pregnancy, postpartum period	
Smoking	
Varicose veins	

Risperidone

Risperidone has also been implicated in cases of antipsychotic-associated pulmonary embolism. Two of the reported cases are from a review of charts in an Emergency Department in Japan and include a 64-year-old woman who had been on risperidone for 40 days and a 48-year-old woman on risperidone for only 6 days [24].

In another case, a 40-year-old man with schizophrenia developed a pulmonary embolism along with rhabdomyolysis 6 weeks after starting a combination of risperidone and mirtazapine [25].

In one case, a 25-year-old man developed a pulmonary embolism on two occasions while being treated with risperidone. Previously, he had developed pulmonary embolism while taking olanzapine [20].

Ziprasidone

Based on premarketing data, the risk of pulmonary embolus with ziprasidone is rare (<0.1%). A search of the literature failed to reveal any independent reports of VTE associated with ziprasidone [26].

First-generation antipsychotic agents

Several case reports, case series, and reviews describing the association between VTE and first-generation antipsychotic use have been published. The risk of VTE appears greatest in the first 3 months of therapy [7,27].

In one case–control study involving patients younger than 60 who had used at least one first- or second-generation antipsychotic agent, exposure to first-generation agents (defined as receipt of an antipsychotic prescription within 60 days preceding the VTE) was associated with a markedly increased risk of VTE compared with non-use (OR 7.1; 95% CI 2.3–22). Although differences among individual agents could not be identified, the group of lower-potency agents (chlorpromazine, thioridazine, mesoridazine, pericyazine, methotrimeprazine, pipotiazine) were associated with a higher risk of VTE than the group of higher-potency agents (haloperidol, pimozide, trifluoperazine, fluphenazine, perphenazine, zuclopenthixol, flupentixol, thiothixene, loxapine) when compared with no antipsychotic (OR = 24.1, 95% CI 3.3–172.7; and OR = 3.3, 95% CI 0.8–13.2, respectively) [27].

In another case–control study comparing cases of fatal pulmonary embolism in patients aged 15–59 with

Table 1.20.2 Signs and symptoms of VTE [2]

Deep-vein thrombosis	Pulmonary embolism
Clinical features:	Clinical features:
Leg pain, tenderness, swelling	Dyspnea, tachypnea
Discoloration (pallor, cyanosis, erythema)	Pleuritic chest pain
Palpable cord (representing a thrombosed vessel)	Cough, rales on auscultation
Venous distension	Hemoptysis (occasionally)
Visible superficial veins	Tachycardia
Positive Homans' sign (pain behind knee or calf upon	Preceding DVT
dorsiflexion of the foot; rarely helpful as only 30%	Accentuated pulmonary component of the
of patients with DVT present with a positive	second heart sound
Homans' sign)	Laboratory features:
Laboratory features:	Elevated fibrinogen and factor VIII
Elevated fibrinogen and factor VIII	Increases in leukocyte and platelet counts
Increases in leukocyte and platelet counts	Systemic activation of blood coagulation, fibrin formation,
Systemic activation of blood coagulation, fibrin formation,	and fibrin breakdown
and fibrin breakdown	Positive D-dimer (fibrin breakdown product)
Positive D-dimer (fibrin breakdown product)	

Monitoring schedule for **ANTIPSYCHOTIC-INDUCED VENOUS THROMBOEMBOLISM (VTE)**

Monitoring includes assessment of pre-existing, new-onset, or changes in risk factors or symptoms of VTE. If the patient has a major risk factor or several minor risk factors, assess for signs and symptoms (present or recent past) of VTE.

	Baseline	Weeks		Months					Long-term monitoring
		1	2	1	2	3	6	12	
Second-generation antipsychotics									
Aripiprazole	•								⭐
Clozapine	•								⭐
Olanzapine	•								⭐
Paliperidone	•								⭐
Quetiapine	•								⭐
Risperidone	•								⭐
Ziprasidone	•								⭐
First-generation antipsychotics									
Chlorpromazine	•								⭐
Flupenthixol	•								⭐
Fluphenazine	•								⭐
Haloperidol	•								⭐
Loxapine	•								⭐
Methotrimeprazine	•								⭐
Molindone	•								⭐
Pericyazine	•								⭐
Perphenazine	•								⭐
Pimozide	•								⭐
Pipotiazine palmitate	•								⭐
Thioridazine	•								⭐
Thiothixene	•								⭐
Trifluoperazine	•								⭐
Zuclopenthixol	•								⭐

• Monitor for adverse effects. ⭐ As clinically indicated.

matched controls, the use of low-potency antipsychotic agents was again associated with a markedly increased risk (OR = 20.8, 95% CI 1.7–259). In this analysis, thioridazine was the low-potency antipsychotic taken in all cases ($n = 7$) of fatal pulmonary embolism observed in patients not known to be at risk of VTE [28].

Monitoring

Prior to the initiation of an antipsychotic agent, patients should be assessed for a history of VTE and risk factors should be reviewed (Table 1.20.1).

Venous thromboembolism should be suspected and investigated appropriately in patients presenting with signs and symptoms suggestive of VTE (see Table 1.20.2), especially if sudden in onset and if antipsychotic treatment is relatively new.

The clinical features of DVT and pulmonary embolism are non-specific, and accurate and timely diagnosis can be challenging but is essential. If VTE is suspected, objective diagnostic laboratory tests and imaging studies are indicated immediately.

REFERENCES

1. Bates SM, Ginsberg JS. Clinical practice. Treatment of deep-vein thrombosis. *N Engl J Med* 2004;**351**(3):268–77.
2. Raskob GE, Hull DH, Pineo GF. Venous thrombosis. In Lichtman MA, Kipps TJ, Kaushansky K, Beutler E, Seligsohn U, Prchal JT, eds., *Williams Hematology*, 7th edn. New York: McGraw-Hill, Medical Publishing Division; 2006.
3. Goldhaber SZ. Pulmonary embolism. *Lancet* 2004;**363**(9417):1295–305.
4. Motykie GD, Zebala LP, Caprini JA, et al. A guide to venous thromboembolism risk factor assessment. *J Thromb Thrombolysis* 2000;**9**(3):253–62.
5. Rosendaal FR. Risk factors for venous thrombotic disease. *Thromb Haemost* 1999;**82**(2):610–19.
6. Douketis JD. Prognosis in pulmonary embolism. *Curr Opin Pulm Med* 2001;**7**(5):354–9.
7. Hagg S, Spigset O. Antipsychotic-induced venous thromboembolism: a review of the evidence. *CNS Drugs* 2002;**16**(11):765–76.
8. Allison DB, Mentore JL, Heo M, et al. Antipsychotic-induced weight gain: a comprehensive research synthesis. *Am J Psychiatry* 1999;**156**(11):1686–96.
9. Greaves M. Antiphospholipid antibodies and thrombosis. *Lancet* 1999;**353**(9161):1348–53.
10. Schwartz M, Rochas M, Weller B, et al. High association of anticardiolipin antibodies with psychosis. *J Clin Psychiatry* 1998;**59**(1):20–3.
11. Lacut K, Le Gal G, Couturaud F, et al. Association between antipsychotic drugs, antidepressant drugs and venous thromboembolism: results from the EDITH case–control study. *Fundam Clin Pharmacol* 2007;**21**(6):643–50.
12. Turpie AGG. Cardiovascular disorders: venous thromboembolism. In Gray J, ed., *Therapeutic Choices*, 5th edn. Ottawa, ON: Canadian Pharmacists Association; 2007.
13. Hagg S, Tatting P, Spigset O. Olanzapine and venous thromboembolism. *Int Clin Psychopharmacol* 2003;**18**(5):299–300.
14. Bristol-Myers Squibb, Otsuka America Pharmaceutical. *Abilify (Aripiprazole) U.S. Full Prescribing Information.* Tokyo, Japan: Otsuka Pharmaceutical Co., Ltd.; 2008.
15. Hagg S, Spigset O, Soderstrom TG. Association of venous thromboembolism and clozapine. *Lancet* 2000;**355**(9210):1155–6.
16. Paciullo CA. Evaluating the association between clozapine and venous thromboembolism. *Am J Health Syst Pharm* 2008;**65**(19):1825–9.
17. Knudson JF, Kortepeter C, Dubitsky GM, Ahmad SR, Chen M. Antipsychotic drugs and venous thromboembolism. *Lancet* 2000;**356**(9225):252–3.
18. Waage IM, Gedde-Dahl A. Pulmonary embolism possibly associated with olanzapine treatment. *BMJ* 2003;**327**(7428):1384.
19. Maly R, Masopust J, Hosak L, Urban A. Four cases of venous thromboembolism associated with olanzapine. *Psychiatry Clin Neurosci* 2009;**63**(1):116–18.
20. Borras L, Eytan A, de Timary P, Constant EL, Huguelet P, Hermans C. Pulmonary thromboembolism associated with olanzapine and risperidone. *J Emerg Med* 2008;**35**(2):159–61.
21. del Conde I, Goldhaber SZ. Pulmonary embolism associated with olanzapine. *Thromb Haemost* 2006;**96**(5):690–1.
22. Toki S, Morinobu S, Yoshino A, Yamawaki S. A case of venous thromboembolism probably associated with hyperprolactinemia after the addition of olanzapine to typical antipsychotics. *J Clin Psychiatry* 2004;**65**(11):1576–7.
23. Janssen-Ortho Inc. *Invega (Paliperidone) Canadian Product Monograph.* Toronto, Canada: Janssen-Ortho Inc.; 2009.
24. Kamijo Y, Soma K, Nagai T, Kurihara K, Ohwada T. Acute massive pulmonary thromboembolism associated with

risperidone and conventional phenothiazines. *Circ J* 2003;**67**(1):46–8.

25. Zink M, Knopf U, Argiriou S, Kuwilsky A. A case of pulmonary thromboembolism and rhabdomyolysis during therapy with mirtazapine and risperidone. *J Clin Psychiatry* 2006;**67**(5):835.

26. Pfizer Canada Inc. *Zeldox (Ziprasidone hydrochloride) Canadian Product Monograph*. Quebec, Canada: Pfizer Canada Inc.; 2007.

27. Zornberg GL, Jick H. Antipsychotic drug use and risk of first-time idiopathic venous thromboembolism: a case–control study. *Lancet* 2000;**356**(9237):1219–23.

28. Parkin L, Skegg DC, Herbison GP, Paul C. Psychotropic drugs and fatal pulmonary embolism. *Pharmacoepidemiol Drug Saf* 2003;**12**(8):647–52.

Vital signs

Background

Measurement of heart rate, blood pressure, core body temperature, and respiratory rate are time-honored means of detecting physiological change. Antipsychotic medications, through multiple direct and indirect effects, can influence these basic measures. Many of the effects are on the cardiocirculatory system. These effects are very common and vary greatly in their significance. They may be dose dependent and many effects are phase dependent with development of tolerance and habituation over time [1].

The effects of antipsychotics on the cardiovascular system are complex due to their direct effects on heart and blood vessels and indirect actions via the central nervous system and autonomic reflexes. Table 1.21.1 gives binding affinities to the relevant receptors. The following pharmacological actions are presumably linked to observed changes in vital signs [1–3]:

Direct effects:
- Peripheral muscarinic anticholinergic effects
- α_1-Adrenoceptor antagonism
- Effects on sodium, potassium, and calcium channels, and on calmodulin

Indirect effects:
- α_2-Adrenoceptors in the central nervous tissue
- Observed effects without known mechanism, such as polyserositis, or myocarditis

Life expectancy is reduced by 20% in people with schizophrenia compared with the general population, with cardiovascular and respiratory illnesses identified as leading causes of death. Social determinants such as poverty and lifestyle issues, including smoking and inactivity, are probable contributory factors [4–6].

Antipsychotics have increasingly been recognized to cause weight gain, to mediate insulin resistance, and to affect lipid metabolism (see Chapters 1.4, 1.5, and 1.9). These disorders may alter physiological functions that are detectable by monitoring vital signs.

Incidents of sudden death have been reported with antipsychotic use since the 1960s. The quinidine-like effects of phenothiazines were initially thought to be protective. Later studies of antiarrhythmic drugs with similar actions showed an increased risk of death in patients taking these drugs [7,8].

All antipsychotics can cause changes in cardiovascular function, although this varies markedly based on the agent's specific pharmacological profile. These effects include tachycardia, postural hypotension, palpitations, arrhythmias, and heart failure, and range in frequency from very common to very rare. High-potency first-generation drugs, such as haloperidol, have fewer anticholinergic and adrenergic α_1 effects and may be more suitable in cases of specific cardiovascular risk [1].

High-dose antipsychotic use has been associated with higher risk for sudden death. More frequent monitoring of vital signs and electrocardiogram (ECG) monitoring is indicated in patients prescribed high doses (see Chapter 1.12) [8–10].

Tachycardia

Anticholinergic effects on the heart are mediated through muscarinic M_2 receptors, which regulate vagal inhibition. Antipsychotic-related M_2 antagonism leads to tachycardia.

Table 1.21.1 Receptor binding affinities of antipsychotics[a] [3]

	α_1	α_2	Muscarinic cholinergic	Histamine H_1	Dopamine D_2	Serotonin 5-HT_2
Aripiprazole	57	–	>10 000	61	0.34	3.4
Chlorpromazine	0.6	750	60	9.1	19	1.4
Clozapine	9	160	7.5	2.7	180	1.6
Flupenthixol	–	–	–	–	–	–
Fluphenazine	9.0	1 600	2 000	21	0.80	19
Haloperidol	6.2	3 800	>20 000	1 890	4	36
Loxapine	28	2 400	62	5	71	1.7
Methotrimeprazine	–	–	–	–	–	–
Molindone	2 500	625	–	>10 000	125	5 000
Olanzapine	19	230	1.9	7.1	11	4
Paliperidone	–	–	–	–	–	–
Pericyazine	–	–	–	–	–	–
Perphenazine	10	510	1 500	–	1.40	5.60
Pimozide	–	–	–	–	2.5	13
Pipotiazine palmitate	–	–	–	–	–	–
Quetiapine	62	2 500	120	11	160	294
Risperidone	2	56	>10 000	59	3.3	0.16
Thioridazine	1.1	–	10	–	2.3	41
Thiothixene (*cis*)	11	200	2 500	6	0.4	130
Trifluoperazine	–	–	–	–	–	–
Ziprasidone	10	260	>10 000	47	0.42	0.42
Zuclopenthixol	–	–	–	–	–	–

[a] Data are inhibitory constant (K_i) values. Lower values indicate higher affinities. Clinical correlates of receptor blockade include (i) adrenergic α_1 receptors: orthostatic hypotension, rebound tachycardia, dizziness, drowsiness; (ii) adrenergic α_2 receptors: putative antidepressant action; (iii) muscarinic receptors: increased heart rate and other anticholinergic effects; (iv) histamine H_1 receptors: weight gain, sedation.

While this is common with clozapine, and frequent with olanzapine and low-potency first-generation drugs, it is regarded as a benign phenomenon in patients with otherwise normal heart function. Tolerance tends to develop with prolonged regular use. Increased heart rate may increase myocardial oxygen demand. In patients with compromised cardiac function, caution is advised [1].

Reduced heart rate variability

Several studies have shown reduced heart rate variability to be a risk factor for cardiac arrhythmias and sudden death in people with heart disease. A reduction in heart rate variability has been observed in people with schizophrenia, independent of pharmacotherapy, as well as with clozapine, thioridazine and fluphenazine. Amisulpride, olanzapine, and risperidone do not appear to adversely affect heart rate variability. Data regarding other agents are unavailable [11–16].

Hypotension

Reduced blood pressure with associated symptoms of feeling faint or weak is a common occurrence with many antipsychotics. Syncopal episodes related to orthostasis are unusual but of concern. Low-potency first-generation antipsychotics are generally considered more likely to cause hypotension and related adverse effects than high-potency selective dopamine antagonists such as haloperidol. α_1-Adrenergic blockade is generally thought to account for this adverse effect, although other putative mechanisms, such as calcium blockade, inhibition of centrally mediated pressor reflexes, and negative inotropic effects, have been proposed [2].

Posture-related drops in blood pressure are especially common with first-generation antipsychotics. Rates as high as 77% have been reported with these agents compared with 15% with placebo. However, this can also be a problem with second-generation agents. A slower dosage titration was recommended when it was observed that the original dosing recommendations for risperidone were frequently associated with postural hypotension and occasionally with fainting. Potent blockade of adrenergic α_1 receptors, which are required for mediating vasoconstriction in certain vascular beds, leads to vasodilation and a rapid blood pressure drop when switching to the standing position. With most drugs, tolerance develops with continued use, and the effects recede [17].

Hypertension

Increases in blood pressure have been reported sporadically, mostly involving clozapine and with the concomitant use of selective serotonin reuptake inhibitors (SSRIs). Other antipsychotics have been implicated very rarely [18].

The New Zealand Intensive Medicines Monitoring Programmme reported 13 cases of hypertension (10 with clozapine, 2 with risperidone, and 1 with quetiapine) compared with 19 cases of presumed hypotension (e.g. faintness) drawn from a sample of 572 case reports. Blood pressure rose sharply shortly after starting the antipsychotic [19].

Temperature and heat dysregulation

Thermoregulation is a complex physiological process that is primarily under the control of hypothalamic temperature-sensitive neurons that prompt autonomic, somatic, and behavioral responses to promote heat conservation or dissipation. Several neurotransmitters and neuropeptides appear to be involved in hypothalamic thermoregulation (e.g. dopamine, serotonin, norepinephrine, acetylcholine, prostaglandins, β-endorphins, neurotensin, intrinsic hypothalamic peptides) [20].

Thermal regulation appears to be altered in schizophrenia and can be compounded by antipsychotic use. Chlorpromazine and other phenothiazines have long been known to affect central thermoregulation resulting in either hypothermia or hyperthermia, depending on the ambient temperature. Based on spontaneous reports involving other antipsychotics, it appears that virtually all antipsychotics can cause this effect with no clear evidence as to which causes it more or less often. The mechanism of this poikilothermic effect is unclear, but is likely mediated by the hypothalamus [21,22].

Impaired body temperature regulation was observed in a controlled trial involving eight patients with schizophrenia taking first-generation intramuscular depot antipsychotics (i.e. haloperidol and fluphenazine) and eight healthy controls. At baseline, skin temperature in the patient group was significantly lower than the healthy controls (33.0 °C vs. 35.3 °C, $p = 0.01$) whereas rectal temperatures were identical. Following an exercise heat tolerance test in a very warm environment, skin temperatures matched (~37.2 °C) but rectal temperature was significantly higher in the patient group (~38.4 °C vs. ~37.8 °C, $p < 0.001$). It was not possible to differentiate between the influences of the drug vs. illness on temperature in this study [23].

An early observation about chlorpromazine as a pre-anesthetic, pre-dating the recognition of its antipsychotic effects, was its ability to suppress the body's natural response to cooling including vasoconstriction and shivering. Chlorpromazine and other antipsychotics may interfere with normal temperature regulation via anticholinergic effects (reduced sweating and heat elimination leading to hyperthermia in warm weather or during exercise) and α-adrenergic antagonist effects (peripheral vasodilation and inhibition of shivering leading to hypothermia in cold weather) [20–22].

A review of antipsychotic-associated hypothermia found 480 reports in the World Health Organization

(WHO) database, which nearly equaled the number of hyperthermia reports. Among the 32 published case reports of 43 people, approximately half involved second-generation antipsychotics. From this study, serotonin 5-HT$_{2a}$ antagonism, a pharmacological feature of most second-generation agents, was also identified as a putative risk factor for antipsychotic-induced hypothermia [22].

The most serious form of thermal dysregulation caused by antipsychotics is neuroleptic malignant syndrome, which is discussed in detail in Chapter 1.8.

Respiratory function

While antipsychotics, or combinations of antipsychotics and other agents, can depress respiratory rate in acute situations (e.g. intramuscular olanzapine and lorazepam combination), respiratory rate is not usually monitored in routine outpatient practice in long-term follow-up of patients.

Agents of interest

The anticholinergic effects of low-potency, first-generation antipsychotics as well as clozapine and olanzapine are detailed in Chapter 1.3.

Second-generation antipsychotic agents

Aripiprazole

A low rate of postural hypotension has been reported with aripiprazole. In short-term, placebo-controlled trials, the incidence of postural hypotension was 1.1% compared with 0.4% on placebo. Postural dizziness and syncope were similar to placebo (0.5% and 0.4%, respectively, with aripiprazole compared with 0.3% and 0.5% with placebo) [24].

Like other antipsychotics, aripiprazole appears to cause hypothermia rarely [22].

Clozapine

Tachycardia was reported in 25% of 842 patients enrolled in clinical trials. The average increase in rate is 10–15 beats per minute. Clinical experience would suggest that

this effect is even more common and is usually transient with cautious dosing increases [25].

Postural hypotension occurs most often during initiation or upward dose titration, but for some patients it is an ongoing phenomenon. In rare instances, this may be catastrophic, accompanied by either respiratory or cardiac arrest. It is advised that if there is treatment interruption of even a very short interval (e.g. 2 days or longer), treatment be reinitiated at a much lower dose [25].

Both hypotension and hypertension have been reported with continued use of clozapine [25].

Ten out of 13 spontaneous reports to the New Zealand Intensive Medicines Monitoring Programmme of antipsychotic-related hypertension implicated clozapine [19].

A chart review of 478 cases from Germany in the 1970s revealed higher rates of hyperthermia with clozapine compared with other antipsychotics (clozapine 15.2%, perazine 3.2%, haloperidol 2.8%). In most cases (83%), hyperthermia occurred within the first 2 weeks of clozapine therapy. While hyperthermia is usually benign with clozapine, neuroleptic malignant syndrome must be ruled out (see Chapter 1.8) [26].

Myocarditis appears to be a rare, potentially fatal risk of clozapine treatment with symptoms of heart failure beginning early in the course of therapy. With a median onset of 2–3 weeks, patient presentation is non-specific and highly variable, and can include tachycardia, shortness of breath, fatigue, cough, chest pain, leukocytosis, and fever. As the presentation is often non-specific, a high index of suspicion, especially within the first 1–2 months, is needed to trigger an ECG and other investigations. Several health regulators, including the US Food and Drug Administration (FDA) and Health Canada, have issued warnings of this risk [27,28].

Like other antipsychotics, clozapine appears to cause hypothermia rarely [22].

Olanzapine

Tachycardia, orthostatic hypotension (>30 mmHg drop in systolic blood pressure), and syncope have been reported with olanzapine at rates of 4% (placebo 1%), 5% (placebo 2%), and 0.6%, respectively [29].

Like other antipsychotics, olanzapine appears to cause hypothermia rarely [22].

Paliperidone

Tachycardia, orthostatic hypotension, and syncope have been reported with paliperidone at rates of 7% (placebo 3%), 2.5% (placebo 0.8%), and 1% (placebo <1%), respectively [30].

Quetiapine

Tachycardia, orthostatic hypotension, and syncope have been reported with immediate-release quetiapine at rates of 7% (placebo 5%), 8% (placebo 2%), and 1% (placebo 0.3%), respectively. These low rates were slightly lower and almost indistinguishable from placebo for the extended-release formulation of quetiapine. The rates with this formulation were 2–3% (0–1% placebo), 3–7% (0–5% placebo), and 0.5% (0.3% placebo), respectively [31,32].

The New Zealand Intensive Medicines Monitoring Programmme reported a single case of treatment-related hypertension involving quetiapine [19].

Like other antipsychotics, quetiapine appears to cause hypothermia rarely [22].

Risperidone

Risperidone has been associated with a dose- and dosing rate-dependent risk of hypotension and tachycardia. Lower initial doses and a slower upward titration rate are now recommended compared with the manufacturer's initial suggestions [33].

In clinical trials, 1.2% discontinued treatment due to cardiovascular side effects including hypotension, tachycardia, and palpitations [33].

Tachycardia, orthostatic hypotension, and syncope have been reported with risperidone at rates of 1–2% (placebo ≤0.5%), 8% (placebo 2%), and 1% (placebo 0.3%), respectively. With the long-acting intramuscular formulation of risperidone, the rates of orthostatic hypotension and syncope were 2% and 0.8% in repeated dose studies [33,34].

Two cases of hypertension were reported to the New Zealand Intensive Medicines Monitoring Programmme.

Elevated blood pressure was observed soon after starting treatment in patients with histories of hypertension. In both cases, an SSRI was concurrently prescribed. Blood pressure returned to normal hours after withdrawal of risperidone [19].

Like other antipsychotics, risperidone appears to cause hypothermia rarely, but possibly more often than other antipsychotics [22].

Ziprasidone

Tachycardia, postural hypotension, and syncope have been reported with ziprasidone at rates of 2% (placebo 1%), 1% (placebo 0%), and 0.6%, respectively [35].

Like other antipsychotics, ziprasidone appears to cause hypothermia rarely [22].

First-generation antipsychotic agents

Chlorpromazine and other low-potency dopamine D_2 antagonists

Chlorpromazine is a low-potency dopamine D_2 antagonist with relatively high affinity for blocking several other receptors, including muscarinic, α-adrenergic, and histaminic receptors (see Table 1.21.1). These effects are shared by other so-called low-potency first-generation antipsychotics such as thioridazine and methotrimeprazine. Thioridazine, mesoridazine,

Table 1.21.2 Vital signs and clinical inquiry

Patients should be asked if they have experienced:	Assessment of vitals should include:
Fever or sweats	Blood pressure (lying and standing)
Pounding heart	
Rapid or jerky heart beat	Heart rate
Dizziness	Pulse pattern (regular, irregular) and volume
Fainting spells or blackouts	
Feeling too hot or cold	Core body temperature (if indicated)
Fatigue, shortness of breath, cough, chest pain (in first 2 months of clozapine treatment)	

Monitoring schedule for **VITAL SIGNS**

Monitoring of vitals is to include, at a minimum, blood pressure, heart rate, and pulse rhythm and volume. Assessment of an orthostatic drop in blood pressure and core body temperature should be based on responses to the clinical inquiry. Refer to other chapters (e.g. Chapters 1.6, 1.9, 1.12) for details regarding other components of the recommended physical assessment of patients taking antipsychotics.

	Baseline	Weeks		Months					Long-term monitoring
		1	2	1	2	3	6	12	
Second-generation antipsychotics									
Aripiprazole	•	•		•		•	•	•	★ ⑥
Clozapine	•ᵃ	•ᵃ	•ᵃ	•ᵃ	•ᵃ	•	•	•	★ ⑥
Olanzapine	•	•		•		•	•	•	★ ⑥
Paliperidone	•	•		•		•	•	•	★ ⑥
Quetiapine	•	•		•		•	•	•	★ ⑥
Risperidone	•	•		•		•	•	•	★ ⑥
Ziprasidone	•	•		•		•	•	•	★ ⑥
First-generation antipsychotics									
Chlorpromazine	•	•		•	•	•	•	•	★ ⑥
Flupenthixol	•	•		•		•	•	•	★ ⑥
Fluphenazine	•	•		•		•	•	•	★ ⑥
Haloperidol	•	•		•		•	•	•	★ ⑥
Loxapine	•	•		•		•	•	•	★ ⑥
Methotrimeprazine	•	•	•	•	•	•	•	•	★ ⑥
Molindone	•	•		•		•	•	•	★ ⑥
Pericyazine	•	•		•		•	•	•	★ ⑥
Perphenazine	•	•		•		•	•	•	★ ⑥
Pimozide	•	•		•		•	•	•	★ ⑥
Pipotiazine palmitate	•	•		•		•	•	•	★ ⑥
Thioridazine	•	•	•	•	•	•	•	•	★ ⑥
Thiothixene	•	•		•		•	•	•	★ ⑥
Trifluoperazine	•	•		•		•	•	•	★ ⑥
Zuclopenthixol	•	•		•		•	•	•	★ ⑥

• Monitor for adverse effect. ★ As clinically indicated. ⑥ Every 6 months.

ᵃ The initiation of clozapine requires intensive monitoring of vital signs due to the high risk of hypotension, tachycardia, and fever. At minimum, blood pressure (including assessment of orthostatic changes), heart rate, pulse, and temperature should be monitored every 2 days during weeks 1 and 2, twice weekly for weeks 3 and 4, and weekly for weeks 5–8. Many centers have more stringent monitoring policies for clozapine initiations.

and other low-potency agents also have common quinidine-like effects on cardiac rhythm [3].

Tachycardia, postural hypotension, hypotension, and syncope are well-known adverse effects of these antipsychotics and are especially problematic with rapid dose escalation.

Temperature dysregulation (e.g. hypothermia, hyperthermia) has long been associated with chlorpromazine, other phenothiazines, and other first-generation antipsychotics. An examination of the WHO international database for Adverse Drug Reactions revealed a statistically increased risk of hypothermia with many commonly used first-generation agents, although the absolute risk appears low [22].

Haloperidol and other high-potency D$_2$ antagonists

Haloperidol is the high-potency dopamine D$_2$ antagonist prototype; however, numerous other first-generation antipsychotics also demonstrate potent antagonistic effects at D$_2$ receptors. These agents tend to have lower affinities for other types of receptors compared with low-potency antipsychotics.

The risk of tachycardia, postural hypotension, hypotension and syncope is lower with high-potency first-generation antipsychotics compared with low-potency agents making them better suited (e.g. haloperidol) for treating medically ill or delirious patients [3].

Similar to low-potency agents, temperature dysregulation presenting as hypothermia or hyperthermia is an uncommon adverse effect [22].

Monitoring

Monitoring of vitals should be a routine component of the patient's treatment assessment.

Clinical inquiries should be used to guide which vital signs should be monitored and how often on an individual basis.

The recommendations provided here are for the average person. Adjustment to the intensity of monitoring should be done on an individual basis depending on past experiences with antipsychotics and other medications, presence or history of other physical conditions (e.g. hypertension, arrhythmias), use of other medications (e.g. hypotensive agents, anticholinergics), and initial effects of the new antipsychotic treatment course.

A complementary clinical inquiry should be a part of the assessment of vitals (Table 1.21.2).

REFERENCES

1. Buckley NA, Sanders P. Cardiovascular adverse effects of antipsychotic drugs. *Drug Saf* 2000;**23**(3):215–28.
2. Fayek M, Kingsbury SJ, Zada J, Simpson GM. Cardiac effects of antipsychotic medications. *Psychiatr Serv* 2001;**52**(5):607–9.
3. Baldessarini RJ, Tarazi FI. Pharmacotherapy of psychosis and mania. In Brunton LL, Lazo JS, Parker K, eds., *Goodman & Gilman's The Pharmacological Basis of Therapeutics*, 11th edn. New York: McGraw-Hill; 2006.
4. Newman SC, Bland RC. Mortality in a cohort of patients with schizophrenia: a record linkage study. *Can J Psychiatry* 1991;**36**(4):239–45.
5. Waddington JL, Youssef HA, Kinsella A. Mortality in schizophrenia. Antipsychotic polypharmacy and absence of adjunctive anticholinergics over the course of a 10-year prospective study. *Br J Psychiatry* 1998;**173**:325–9.
6. Seeman MV. An outcome measure in schizophrenia: mortality. *Can J Psychiatry* 2007;**52**(1):55–60.
7. Haddad PM, Anderson IM. Antipsychotic-related QTc prolongation, torsade de pointes and sudden death. *Drugs* 2002;**62**(11):1649–71.
8. Ray WA, Chung CP, Murray KT, Hall K, Stein CM. Atypical antipsychotic drugs and the risk of sudden cardiac death. *N Engl J Med* 2009;**360**(3):225–35.
9. Ray WA, Meredith S, Thapa PB, Meador KG, Hall K, Murray KT. Antipsychotics and the risk of sudden cardiac death. *Arch Gen Psychiatry* 2001;**58**(12):1161–7.
10. Straus SM, Bleumink GS, Dieleman JP, et al. Antipsychotics and the risk of sudden cardiac death. *Arch Intern Med* 2004;**164**(12):1293–7.
11. Huikuri HV, Makikallio T, Airaksinen KE, Mitrani R, Castellanos A, Myerburg RJ. Measurement of heart rate variability: a clinical tool or a research toy? *J Am Coll Cardiol* 1999;**34**(7):1878–83.

12. Agelink MW, Malessa R, Kamcili E, et al. Cardiovascular autonomic reactivity in schizophrenics under neuroleptic treatment: a potential predictor of short-term outcome? *Neuropsychobiology* 1998;**38**(1):19–24.

13. Zahn TP, Pickar D. Autonomic effects of clozapine in schizophrenia: comparison with placebo and fluphenazine. *Biol Psychiatry* 1993;**34**(1–2):3–12.

14. Silke B, Campbell C, King DJ. The potential cardiotoxicity of antipsychotic drugs as assessed by heart rate variability. *J Psychopharmacol* 2002;**16**(4):355–60.

15. Wang YC, Yang CC, Bai YM, Kuo TB. Heart rate variability in schizophrenic patients switched from typical antipsychotic agents to amisulpride and olanzapine. 3-Month follow-up. *Neuropsychobiology* 2008;**57**(4):200–5.

16. Stein KM. Noninvasive risk stratification for sudden death: signal-averaged electrocardiography, nonsustained ventricular tachycardia, heart rate variability, baroreflex sensitivity, and QRS duration. *Prog Cardiovasc Dis* 2008;**51**(2):106–17.

17. Silver H, Kogan H, Zlotogorski D. Postural hypotension in chronically medicated schizophrenics. *J Clin Psychiatry* 1990;**51**(11):459–62.

18. Ennis LM, Parker RM. Paradoxical hypertension associated with clozapine. *Med J Aust* 1997;**166**(5):278.

19. Coulter D. Atypical antipsychotics may cause hypotension. *Prescriber Update* 2003;**24**(1):4–5.

20. Vassallo SU, Delany KA. Thermoregulatory principles. In Wonsiewicz MJ, Edmonson KG, Boyle PJ, eds., *Goldfrank's Toxicologic Emergencies*, 8th edn. New York: McGraw Hill; 2006.

21. Martinez M, Devenport L, Saussy J, Martinez J. Drug-associated heat stroke. *South Med J* 2002;**95**(8):799–802.

22. van Marum RJ, Wegewijs MA, Loonen AJ, Beers E. Hypothermia following antipsychotic drug use. *Eur J Clin Pharmacol* 2007;**63**(6):627–31.

23. Hermesh H, Shiloh R, Epstein Y, Manaim H, Weizman A, Munitz H. Heat intolerance in patients with chronic schizophrenia maintained with antipsychotic drugs. *Am J Psychiatry* 2000;**157**(8):1327–9.

24. Bristol-Myers Squibb Canada. *Abilify (Aripiprazole) Product Monograph*. Montreal, Canada: Bristol-Myers Squibb Canada; 2009.

25. Novartis Pharmaceuticals Canada Inc. *Clozaril (Clozapine) Canadian Prescribing Information*. Dorval, QC: Novartis Pharmaceuticals Canada Inc.; 2007.

26. Bauer D, Gaertner HJ. Effects of neuroleptics on liver function, the hematopoietic system, blood pressure and temperature regulation. Comparison of clozapine, perazine and haloperidol by evaluating medical records. *Pharmacopsychiatria* 1983;**16**(1):23–9.

27. Layland JJ, Liew D, Prior DL. Clozapine-induced cardiotoxicity: a clinical update. *Med J Aust* 2009;**190**(4):190–2.

28. Haas SJ, Hill R, Krum H, et al. Clozapine-associated myocarditis: a review of 116 cases of suspected myocarditis associated with the use of clozapine in Australia during 1993–2003. *Drug Saf* 2007;**30**(1):47–57.

29. Lilly. *Zyprexa (Olanzapine) Product Monograph*. Toronto, Canada: Lilly; 2008.

30. Janssen-Ortho Inc. *Invega (Paliperidone) Canadian Product Monograph*. Toronto, Canada: Janssen-Ortho Inc.; 2009.

31. AstraZeneca Canada Inc. *Seroquel XR (Quetiapine fumarate) Canadian Product Monograph*. Mississauga, ON: AstraZeneca Canada Inc.; 2009.

32. AstraZeneca Canada Inc. *Seroquel (Quetiapine) Product Monograph*. Toronto, Canada: AstraZeneca Canada Inc.; 2008.

33. Janssen-Ortho Inc. *Risperdal (Risperidone) Product Monograph*. Toronto, Canada: Janssen-Ortho Inc.; 2008.

34. Janssen-Ortho Inc. *Risperdal Consta (Risperidone) Product Monograph*. Toronto, Canada: Janssen-Ortho Inc.; 2009.

35. Pfizer Canada Inc. *Zeldox (Ziprasidone hydrochloride) Canadian Product Monograph*. Quebec, Canada: Pfizer Canada Inc.; 2007.

SECTION 2

Summary of monitoring recommendations for individual antipsychotics

Section 2 consists of individual antipsychotic monitoring schedules recommended for each individual antipsychotic agent. They are organized alphabetically by drug name. Each drug's monitoring schedule is unique and provides clear recommendations regarding what to monitor and when to monitor it. The information in these monitoring recommendations is simply a reorganization of the information provided in the 20 side effect chapters of Section 1. This section of the book will be most useful once the practitioner has selected an antipsychotic for an individual patient and wishes to put a monitoring schedule in place. If unclear about how to monitor any of the listed side effects, refer to the respective chapter in Section 1.

Aripiprazole

Monitoring schedule recommended for **ARIPIPRAZOLE**

For specific monitoring recommendations related to each adverse effect, refer to the monitoring subheading of each chapter in Section 1.

	Baseline	Weeks		Months					Long-term monitoring
		1	2	1	2	3	6	12	
Adverse effect									
Agranulocytosis/blood dyscrasias	•								★
Anticholinergic effects	•	•							★
Diabetes	•						•	•	★ ⑫
Dyslipidemia	•							•	★ ⑫
Extrapyramidal symptoms	•		•	•		•			★ ⑫
Hepatic effects	•			•					★
Neuroleptic malignant syndrome	•								★
Obesity/weight gain	•			•		•	•	•	★ ⑥
Ocular effects	•								★
Prolactin effects	•								★
QT prolongation/arrhythmias	•		•		•		•		★
Sedation/sleep disturbances	•		•	•	•		•		★
Seizures	•								★
Sexual dysfunction	•					•	•	•	★ ⑥
Sialorrhea	•								★
Skin/hypersensitivity reactions	•			•			•		★
Tardive dyskinesia	•						•	•	★ ⑫
Urinary incontinence	•			•					★
Venous thromboembolism	•								★
Vital signs	•	•	•	•		•	•	•	★ ⑥

• Monitor for adverse effect. ★ As clinically indicated. ⑥ Every 6 months. ⑫ Annually.

Notes: _____

_____

_____

Chlorpromazine

Monitoring schedule recommended for **CHLORPROMAZINE**

For specific monitoring recommendations related to each adverse effect, refer to the monitoring subheading of each chapter in Section 1.

	Baseline	Weeks 1	Weeks 2	Months 1	Months 2	Months 3	Months 6	Months 12	Long-term monitoring
Adverse effect									
Agranulocytosis/blood dyscrasias	•								★
Anticholinergic effects	•	•	•	•		•			★
Diabetes	•					•	•	•	★ ⑥
Dyslipidemia	•					•		•	★ ⑫
Extrapyramidal symptoms	•	•	•	•	•	•	•	•	★ ⑥
Hepatic effects	•			•					★
Neuroleptic malignant syndrome	•								★
Obesity/weight gain	•		•	•	•	•	•	•	★ ③
Ocular effects	•						•	•	★ ⑥
Prolactin effects	•				•		•	•	★ ⑥
QT prolongation/arrhythmias	•		•		•		•		★
Sedation/sleep disturbances	•	•	•	•		•			★
Seizures	•					•			★
Sexual dysfunction	•					•		•	★ ⑥
Sialorrhea	•								★
Skin/hypersensitivity reactions	•			•			•		★
Tardive dyskinesia	•					•	•	•	★ ⑥
Urinary incontinence	•			•					★
Venous thromboembolism	•								★
Vital signs	•	•	•	•	•	•	•	•	★ ⑥

• Monitor for adverse effect. ★ As clinically indicated. ③ Every 3 months. ⑥ Every 6 months. ⑫ Annually.

Notes: _____

_____

_____

Clozapine

Monitoring schedule recommended for **CLOZAPINE**

For specific monitoring recommendations related to each adverse effect, refer to the monitoring subheading of each chapter in Section 1.

	Baseline	Weeks		Months					Long-term monitoring
		1	2	1	2	3	6	12	
Adverse effect									
Agranulocytosis/blood dyscrasias^a	•	Weekly × 26 weeks, biweekly × 26 weeks, then every 4 weeks thereafter							(★)
Anticholinergic effects	•	•	•	•	•	•	•	•	(★)
Diabetes	•					•	•	•	(★) (6)
Dyslipidemia	•					•		•	(★) (12)
Extrapyramidal symptoms	•			•		•			(★) (12)
Hepatic effects	•			•					(★)
Neuroleptic malignant syndrome	•								(★)
Obesity/weight gain	•		•	•	•	•	•	•	(★) (3)
Ocular effects	•								(★)
Prolactin effects	•								(★)
QT prolongation/arrhythmias	•		•		•		•		(★)
Sedation/sleep disturbances	•	•	•	•	•	•	•	•	(★)
Seizures	•			•		•			(★)
Sexual dysfunction	•			•		•	•	•	(★) (6)
Sialorrhea^b	•	•	•	•	•	•			(★)
Skin/hypersensitivity reactions	•			•			•		(★)
Tardive dyskinesia	•						•	•	(★) (12)
Urinary incontinence	•		•	•	•	•			(★)
Venous thromboembolism	•								(★)
Vital signs^c	•	•	•	•	•	•	•	•	(★) (6)

• Monitor for adverse effect. (★) As clinically indicated. (3) Every 3 months. (6) Every 6 months. (12) Annually.

^a Complete blood count with differential reporting of neutrophils is required in Canada, the UK, the USA, and numerous other countries. The requirements of monitoring and reporting vary among regulatory authorities. More intensive monitoring is required when leukocyte counts are reduced. Refer to your local requirements for details. Upon discontinuation of clozapine for any reason, monitoring must be continued for 4 weeks.

^b Screen for and assess sialorrhea frequently in the first 6 months; reduce frequency to every 3 months thereafter if not problematic.

^c The initiation of clozapine requires intensive monitoring of vital signs due to the high risk of hypotension, tachycardia, and fever. At minimum, blood pressure (including assessment of orthostatic changes), heart rate, pulse, and temperature should be monitored every 2 days during weeks 1 and 2, twice weekly for weeks 3 and 4, and weekly for weeks 5–8.

Notes: _____

_____

_____

Flupenthixol

Monitoring schedule recommended for **FLUPENTHIXOL**

For specific monitoring recommendations related to each adverse effect, refer to the monitoring subheading of each chapter in Section 1.

	Baseline	Weeks		Months					Long-term monitoring
		1	2	1	2	3	6	12	
Adverse effect									
Agranulocytosis/blood dyscrasias	•								(★)
Anticholinergic effects	•	Δ	•	Δ	Δ				(★)
Diabetes	•						•	•	(★) (12)
Dyslipidemia	•							•	(★) (12)
Extrapyramidal symptoms	•	•	•	•	•	•	•	•	(★) (6)
Hepatic effects	•			•					(★)
Neuroleptic malignant syndrome	•								(★)
Obesity/weight gain	•			•		•			(★) (6)
Ocular effects	•								(★)
Prolactin effects	•				•	•	•	•	(★) (6)
QT prolongation/arrhythmias	•		•		•		•		(★)
Sedation/sleep disturbances	•		•	•	•		•		(★)
Seizures	•								(★)
Sexual dysfunction	•					•		•	(★) (6)
Sialorrhea	•								(★)
Skin/hypersensitivity reactions	•			•			•		(★)
Tardive dyskinesia	•					•	•	•	(★) (6)
Urinary incontinence	•			•					(★)
Venous thromboembolism	•								(★)
Vital signs	•	•		•		•	•	•	(★) (6)

• Monitor for adverse effect. (★) As clinically indicated. (6) Every 6 months. (12) Annually. Δ Additional monitoring is recommended when an anticholinergic agent is co-prescribed with the antipsychotic.

Notes: _____

_____

_____

Fluphenazine

Monitoring schedule recommended for **FLUPHENAZINE**

For specific monitoring recommendations related to each adverse effect, refer to the monitoring subheading of each chapter in Section 1.

	Baseline	Weeks 1	Weeks 2	Months 1	2	3	6	12	Long-term monitoring
Adverse effect									
Agranulocytosis/blood dyscrasias	•								(★)
Anticholinergic effects	•	Δ	•	Δ	Δ				(★)
Diabetes	•						•	•	(★) (12)
Dyslipidemia	•					•		•	(★) (12)
Extrapyramidal symptoms	•	•	•	•	•	•	•	•	(★) (6)
Hepatic effects	•			•					(★)
Neuroleptic malignant syndrome	•								(★)
Obesity/weight gain	•			•		•			(★) (6)
Ocular effects	•						•	•	(★) (6)
Prolactin effects	•			•		•	•	•	(★) (6)
QT prolongation/arrhythmias	•		•		•		•		(★)
Sedation/sleep disturbances	•		•	•	•		•		(★)
Seizures	•								(★)
Sexual dysfunction	•					•	•		(★) (6)
Sialorrhea	•								(★)
Skin/hypersensitivity reactions	•			•			•		(★)
Tardive dyskinesia	•					•	•	•	(★) (6)
Urinary incontinence	•			•					(★)
Venous thromboembolism	•								(★)
Vital signs	•	•		•		•	•	•	(★) (6)

• Monitor for adverse effect. (★) As clinically indicated. (6) Every 6 months. (12) Annually. Δ Additional monitoring is recommended when an anticholinergic agent is co-prescribed with the antipsychotic.

Notes: _____

_____

_____

Haloperidol

Monitoring schedule recommended for **HALOPERIDOL**

For specific monitoring recommendations related to each adverse effect, refer to the monitoring subheading of each chapter in Section 1.

	Baseline	Weeks 1	Weeks 2	Months 1	Months 2	Months 3	Months 6	Months 12	Long-term monitoring
Adverse effect									
Agranulocytosis/blood dyscrasias	•								⊛
Anticholinergic effects	•	Δ	•	Δ	Δ				⊛
Diabetes	•						•	•	⊛ ⑫
Dyslipidemia	•							•	⊛ ⑫
Extrapyramidal symptoms	•	•	•	•	•	•	•	•	⊛ ⑥
Hepatic effects	•			•					⊛
Neuroleptic malignant syndrome	•								⊛
Obesity/weight gain	•			•		•			⊛ ⑥
Ocular effects	•								⊛
Prolactin effects	•			•		•	•	•	⊛ ⑥
QT prolongation/arrhythmias	•		•		•		•		⊛
Sedation/sleep disturbances	•		•	•	•		•		⊛
Seizures	•								⊛
Sexual dysfunction	•				•		•	•	⊛ ⑥
Sialorrhea	•			•					⊛
Skin/hypersensitivity reactions	•			•			•		⊛
Tardive dyskinesia	•				•		•	•	⊛ ⑥
Urinary incontinence	•			•					⊛
Venous thromboembolism	•								⊛
Vital signs	•	•		•		•	•	•	⊛ ⑥

• Monitor for adverse effect. ⊛ As clinically indicated. ⑥ Every 6 months. ⑫ Annually. Δ Additional monitoring is recommended when an anticholinergic agent is co-prescribed with the antipsychotic.

Notes: _____

_____

_____

Loxapine

Monitoring schedule recommended for **LOXAPINE**

For specific monitoring recommendations related to each adverse effect, refer to the monitoring subheading of each chapter in Section 1

	Baseline	Weeks		Months					Long-term monitoring
		1	2	1	2	3	6	12	
Adverse effect									
Agranulocytosis/blood dyscrasias	•								⭐
Anticholinergic effects	•	Δ	•	Δ	Δ				⭐
Diabetes	•						•	•	⭐ ⑫
Dyslipidemia	•							•	⭐ ⑫
Extrapyramidal symptoms	•	•	•	•	•	•		•	⭐ ⑥
Hepatic effects	•			•					⭐
Neuroleptic malignant syndrome	•								⭐
Obesity/weight gain	•			•		•			⭐ ⑥
Ocular effects	•								⭐
Prolactin effects	•			•		•	•	•	⭐ ⑥
QT prolongation/arrhythmias	•		•		•		•		⭐
Sedation/sleep disturbances	•	•	•	•	•		•		⭐
Seizures	•								⭐
Sexual dysfunction	•					•	•	•	⭐ ⑥
Sialorrhea	•								⭐
Skin/hypersensitivity reactions	•			•			•		⭐
Tardive dyskinesia	•					•	•	•	⭐ ⑥
Urinary incontinence	•			•					⭐
Venous thromboembolism	•								⭐
Vital signs	•	•		•		•	•	•	⭐ ⑥

• Monitor for adverse effect. ⭐ As clinically indicated. ⑥ Every 6 months. ⑫ Annually. Δ Additional monitoring is recommended when an anticholinergic agent is co-prescribed with the antipsychotic.

Notes: _____

_____

_____

Methotrimeprazine

Monitoring schedule recommended for **METHOTRIMEPRAZINE**

For specific monitoring recommendations related to each adverse effect, refer to the monitoring subheading of each chapter in Section 1.

	Baseline	Weeks 1	Weeks 2	Months 1	Months 2	Months 3	Months 6	Months 12	Long-term monitoring
Adverse effect									
Agranulocytosis/blood dyscrasias	•								★
Anticholinergic effects	•	•	•	•		•			★
Diabetes	•						•	•	★ ⑫
Dyslipidemia	•					•		•	★ ⑫
Extrapyramidal symptoms	•	•	•	•	•	•	•	•	★ ⑥
Hepatic effects	•				•				★
Neuroleptic malignant syndrome	•								★
Obesity/weight gain	•		•	•	•	•	•	•	★ ③
Ocular effects	•						•	•	★ ⑥
Prolactin effects	•			•		•	•	•	★ ⑥
QT prolongation/arrhythmias	•		•		•		•		★
Sedation/sleep disturbances	•	•	•	•	•		•		★
Seizures	•								★
Sexual dysfunction	•					•	•	•	★ ⑥
Sialorrhea	•								★
Skin/hypersensitivity reactions	•			•			•		★
Tardive dyskinesia	•					•	•	•	★ ⑥
Urinary incontinence	•			•					★
Venous thromboembolism	•								★
Vital signs	•	•	•	•	•	•	•	•	★ ⑥

• Monitor for adverse effect. ★ As clinically indicated. ③ Every 3 months. ⑥ Every 6 months. ⑫ Annually.

Notes: _____

_____

_____

Molindone

Monitoring schedule recommended for **MOLINDONE**

For specific monitoring recommendations related to each adverse effect, refer to the monitoring subheading of each chapter in Section 1.

	Baseline	Weeks		Months					Long-term monitoring
		1	2	1	2	3	6	12	
Adverse effect									
Agranulocytosis/blood dyscrasias	•								ⓐ
Anticholinergic effects	•	Δ	•	Δ	Δ				ⓐ
Diabetes	•						•	•	ⓐ ⑫
Dyslipidemia	•							•	ⓐ ⑫
Extrapyramidal symptoms	•	•	•	•	•	•	•	•	ⓐ ⑥
Hepatic effects	•			•					ⓐ
Neuroleptic malignant syndrome	•								ⓐ
Obesity/weight gain	•			•		•			ⓐ ⑥
Ocular effects	•								ⓐ
Prolactin effects	•			•		•	•	•	ⓐ ⑥
QT prolongation/arrhythmias	•		•		•		•		ⓐ
Sedation/sleep disturbances	•		•	•	•		•		ⓐ
Seizures	•								ⓐ
Sexual dysfunction	•					•	•	•	ⓐ ⑥
Sialorrhea	•								ⓐ
Skin/hypersensitivity reactions	•			•			•		ⓐ
Tardive dyskinesia	•					•	•	•	ⓐ ⑥
Urinary incontinence	•			•					ⓐ
Venous thromboembolism	•								ⓐ
Vital signs	•	•		•		•	•	•	ⓐ ⑥

• Monitor for adverse effect. ⓐ As clinically indicated. ⑥ Every 6 months. ⑫ Annually. Δ Additional monitoring is recommended when an anticholinergic agent is co-prescribed with the antipsychotic.

Notes: _____

_____

_____

Olanzapine

Monitoring schedule recommended for **OLANZAPINE**

For specific monitoring recommendations related to each adverse effect, refer to the monitoring subheading of each chapter in Section 1.

Adverse effect	Baseline	Weeks 1	Weeks 2	Months 1	Months 2	Months 3	Months 6	Months 12	Long-term monitoring
Agranulocytosis/blood dyscrasias	•								⊛
Anticholinergic effects	•			•		•			⊛
Diabetes	•					•	•	•	⊛ ⑥
Dyslipidemia	•					•		•	⊛ ⑫
Extrapyramidal symptoms	•		•	•		•	•	•	⊛ ⑥
Hepatic effects	•			•					⊛
Neuroleptic malignant syndrome	•								⊛
Obesity/weight gain	•		•	•	•	•	•	•	⊛ ③
Ocular effects	•								⊛
Prolactin effects	•								⊛
QT prolongation/arrhythmias	•		•		•		•		⊛
Sedation/sleep disturbances	•		•	•	•		•		⊛
Seizures	•								⊛
Sexual dysfunction	•					•	•	•	⊛ ⑥
Sialorrhea	•								⊛
Skin/hypersensitivity reactions	•			•			•		⊛
Tardive dyskinesia	•						•	•	⊛ ⑫
Urinary incontinence	•			•					⊛
Venous thromboembolism	•								⊛
Vital signs	•	•		•		•	•	•	⊛ ⑥

• Monitor for adverse effect. ⊛ As clinically indicated. ③ Every 3 months. ⑥ Every 6 months. ⑫ Annually.

Notes: _____

Paliperidone

Monitoring schedule recommended for **PALIPERIDONE**

For specific monitoring recommendations related to each adverse effect, refer to the monitoring subheading of each chapter in Section 1.

	Baseline	Weeks		Months					Long-term monitoring
		1	2	1	2	3	6	12	
Adverse effect									
Agranulocytosis/blood dyscrasias	•								(★)
Anticholinergic effects	•	Δ	Δ	Δ	Δ				(★)
Diabetes	•						•	•	(★) (12)
Dyslipidemia	•					•		•	(★) (12)
Extrapyramidal symptoms	•	•	•	•	•	•		•	(★) (6)
Hepatic effects	•			•					(★)
Neuroleptic malignant syndrome	•								(★)
Obesity/weight gain	•		•	•	•	•		•	(★) (6)
Ocular effects	•								(★)
Prolactin effects	•			•		•		•	(★) (6)
QT prolongation/arrhythmias	•		•		•		•		(★)
Sedation/sleep disturbances	•		•	•	•				(★)
Seizures	•								(★)
Sexual dysfunction	•			•		•	•	•	(★) (6)
Sialorrhea	•			•					(★)
Skin/hypersensitivity reactions	•			•			•		(★)
Tardive dyskinesia	•						•	•	(★) (12)
Urinary incontinence	•		•	•	•	•			(★)
Venous thromboembolism	•								(★)
Vital signs	•	•		•		•	•	•	(★) (6)

• Monitor for adverse effect. (★) As clinically indicated. (6) Every 6 months. (12) Annually. Δ Additional monitoring is recommended when an anticholinergic agent is co-prescribed with the antipsychotic.

Notes: _____

_____

_____

2.12

Pericyazine

Monitoring schedule recommended for **PERICYAZINE**

For specific monitoring recommendations related to each adverse effect, refer to the monitoring subheading of each chapter in Section 1.

	Baseline	Weeks 1	Weeks 2	Months 1	Months 2	Months 3	Months 6	Months 12	Long-term monitoring
Adverse effect									
Agranulocytosis/blood dyscrasias	•								(★)
Anticholinergic effects	•	Δ	•	Δ	Δ				(★)
Diabetes	•						•	•	(★) (12)
Dyslipidemia	•					•		•	(★) (12)
Extrapyramidal symptoms	•	•	•	•	•	•	•	•	(★) (6)
Hepatic effects	•			•					(★)
Neuroleptic malignant syndrome	•								(★)
Obesity/weight gain	•			•		•			(★) (6)
Ocular effects	•								(★)
Prolactin effects	•			•		•		•	(★) (6)
QT prolongation/arrhythmias	•		•		•		•		(★)
Sedation/sleep disturbances	•			•	•	•	•		(★)
Seizures	•								(★)
Sexual dysfunction	•					•	•	•	(★) (6)
Sialorrhea	•								(★)
Skin/hypersensitivity reactions	•			•			•		(★)
Tardive dyskinesia	•					•	•	•	(★) (6)
Urinary incontinence	•			•					(★)
Venous thromboembolism	•								(★)
Vital signs	•	•		•		•	•	•	(★) (6)

• Monitor for adverse effect. (★) As clinically indicated. (6) Every 6 months. (12) Annually. Δ Additional monitoring is recommended when an anticholinergic agent is co-prescribed with the antipsychotic.

Notes: _____

_____

_____

Perphenazine

Monitoring schedule recommended for **PERPHENAZINE**

For specific monitoring recommendations related to each adverse effect, refer to the monitoring subheading of each chapter in Section 1.

	Baseline	Weeks 1	Weeks 2	Months 1	Months 2	Months 3	Months 6	Months 12	Long-term monitoring
Adverse effect									
Agranulocytosis/blood dyscrasias	•								⊛
Anticholinergic effects	•	Δ	•	Δ	Δ				⊛
Diabetes	•						•	•	⊛ ⑫
Dyslipidemia	•					•		•	⊛ ⑫
Extrapyramidal symptoms	•	•	•	•	•	•	•	•	⊛ ⑥
Hepatic effects	•			•					⊛
Neuroleptic malignant syndrome	•								⊛
Obesity/weight gain	•		•	•	•	•	•	•	⊛ ③
Ocular effects	•						•	•	⊛ ⑥
Prolactin effects	•			•		•	•	•	⊛ ⑥
QT prolongation/arrhythmias	•		•		•		•		⊛
Sedation/sleep disturbances	•		•	•	•		•		⊛
Seizures	•								⊛
Sexual dysfunction	•					•	•	•	⊛ ⑥
Sialorrhea	•								⊛
Skin/hypersensitivity reactions	•			•			•		⊛
Tardive dyskinesia	•					•	•	•	⊛ ⑥
Urinary incontinence	•			•					⊛
Venous thromboembolism	•								⊛
Vital signs	•	•		•		•	•	•	⊛ ⑥

• Monitor for adverse effect. ⊛ As clinically indicated. ③ Every 3 months. ⑥ Every 6 months. ⑫ Annually. Δ Additional monitoring is recommended when an anticholinergic agent is co-prescribed with the antipsychotic.

Notes: _____

_____

_____

Pimozide

Monitoring schedule recommended for **PIMOZIDE**

For specific monitoring recommendations related to each adverse effect, refer to the monitoring subheading of each chapter in Section 1.

	Baseline	Weeks 1	Weeks 2	Months 1	Months 2	Months 3	Months 6	Months 12	Long-term monitoring
Adverse effect									
Agranulocytosis/blood dyscrasias	•								★
Anticholinergic effects	•	Δ	•	Δ	Δ				★
Diabetes	•						•	•	★ 12
Dyslipidemia	•							•	★ 12
Extrapyramidal symptoms	•	•	•	•	•	•	•	•	★ 6
Hepatic effects	•			•					★
Neuroleptic malignant syndrome	•								★
Obesity/weight gain	•			•		•			★ 6
Ocular effects	•								★
Prolactin effects	•			•		•	•		★ 6
QT prolongation/arrhythmias	•		•		•		•		★
Sedation/sleep disturbances	•		•	•	•		•		★
Seizures	•								★
Sexual dysfunction	•					•	•	•	★ 6
Sialorrhea	•								★
Skin/hypersensitivity reactions	•			•			•		★
Tardive dyskinesia	•					•	•	•	★ 6
Urinary incontinence	•			•					★
Venous thromboembolism	•								★
Vital signs	•	•		•		•	•	•	★ 6

• Monitor for adverse effect. ★ As clinically indicated. ⑥ Every 6 months. ⑫ Annually. Δ Additional monitoring is recommended when an anticholinergic agent is co-prescribed with the antipsychotic.

Notes: _____

_____

_____

Pipotiazine palmitate

Monitoring schedule recommended for **PIPOTIAZINE PALMITATE**

For specific monitoring recommendations related to each adverse effect, refer to the monitoring subheading of each chapter in Section 1.

	Baseline	Weeks 1	Weeks 2	Months 1	Months 2	Months 3	Months 6	Months 12	Long-term monitoring
Adverse effect									
Agranulocytosis/blood dyscrasias	•								★
Anticholinergic effects	•	Δ	•	Δ	Δ				★
Diabetes	•						•	•	★ ⑫
Dyslipidemia	•					•		•	★ ⑫
Extrapyramidal symptoms	•	•	•	•	•	•	•	•	★ ⑥
Hepatic effects	•			•					★
Neuroleptic malignant syndrome	•								★
Obesity/weight gain	•			•		•			★ ⑥
Ocular effects	•								★
Prolactin effects	•			•		•	•	•	★ ⑥
QT prolongation/arrhythmias	•		•		•		•		★
Sedation/sleep disturbances	•		•	•	•		•		★
Seizures	•								★
Sexual dysfunction	•					•	•	•	★ ⑥
Sialorrhea	•								★
Skin/hypersensitivity reactions	•			•			•		★
Tardive dyskinesia	•					•	•	•	★ ⑥
Urinary incontinence	•			•					★
Venous thromboembolism	•								★
Vital signs	•		•	•		•	•	•	★ ⑥

• Monitor for adverse effect. ★ As clinically indicated. ⑥ Every 6 months. ⑫ Annually. Δ Additional monitoring is recommended when an anticholinergic agent is co-prescribed with the antipsychotic.

Notes: _____

_____

_____

Quetiapine

Monitoring schedule recommended for **QUETIAPINE**

For specific monitoring recommendations related to each adverse effect, refer to the monitoring subheading of each chapter in Section 1.

	Baseline	Weeks 1	Weeks 2	Months 1	2	3	6	12	Long-term monitoring
Adverse effect									
Agranulocytosis/blood dyscrasias	•								(★)
Anticholinergic effects	•			•		•			(★)
Diabetes	•						•	•	(★) (12)
Dyslipidemia	•					•		•	(★) (12)
Extrapyramidal symptoms	•			•		•			(★) (12)
Hepatic effects	•			•					(★)
Neuroleptic malignant syndrome	•								(★)
Obesity/weight gain	•		•	•	•	•	•	•	(★) (3)
Ocular effects	•								(★)
Prolactin effects	•								(★)
QT prolongation/arrhythmias	•		•		•		•		(★)
Sedation/sleep disturbances	•		•	•	•		•		(★)
Seizures	•								(★)
Sexual dysfunction	•					•	•	•	(★) (6)
Sialorrhea	•								(★)
Skin/hypersensitivity reactions	•			•			•		(★)
Tardive dyskinesia	•						•	•	(★) (12)
Urinary incontinence	•			•					(★)
Venous thromboembolism	•								(★)
Vital signs	•	•		•		•	•	•	(★) (6)

• Monitor for adverse effect. (★) As clinically indicated. (3) Every 3 months. (6) Every 6 months. (12) Annually.

Notes: _____

_____

_____

Risperidone

Monitoring schedule recommended for **RISPERIDONE**

For specific monitoring recommendations related to each adverse effect, refer to the monitoring subheading of each chapter in Section 1.

	Baseline	Weeks		Months					Long-term monitoring
		1	2	1	2	3	6	12	
Adverse effect									
Agranulocytosis/blood dyscrasias	•								⊛
Anticholinergic effects	•	Δ	Δ	Δ	Δ				⊛
Diabetes	•						•	•	⊛ ⑫
Dyslipidemia	•					•		•	⊛ ⑫
Extrapyramidal symptoms	•	•	•	•	•	•	•	•	⊛ ⑥
Hepatic effects	•			•					⊛
Neuroleptic malignant syndrome	•								⊛
Obesity/weight gain	•		•	•	•	•	•	•	⊛ ③
Ocular effects	•								⊛
Prolactin effects	•			•		•	•	•	⊛ ⑥
QT prolongation/arrhythmias	•		•		•		•		⊛
Sedation/sleep disturbances	•		•	•	•		•		⊛
Seizures	•								⊛
Sexual dysfunction	•			•		•	•	•	⊛ ⑥
Sialorrhea	•			•					⊛
Skin/hypersensitivity reactions	•			•			•		⊛
Tardive dyskinesia	•						•	•	⊛ ⑫
Urinary incontinence	•		•	•	•	•			⊛
Venous thromboembolism	•								⊛
Vital signs	•	•		•		•	•	•	⊛ ⑥

• Monitor for adverse effect. ⊛ As clinically indicated. ③ Every 3 months. ⑥ Every 6 months. ⑫ Annually. Δ Additional monitoring is recommended when an anticholinergic agent is co-prescribed with the antipsychotic.

Notes: _____

_____

_____

_____

2.18

Thioridazine

Monitoring schedule recommended for **THIORIDAZINE**

For specific monitoring recommendations related to each adverse effect, refer to the monitoring subheading of each chapter in Section 1.

		Weeks		Months					
	Baseline	1	2	1	2	3	6	12	Long-term monitoring
Adverse effect									
Agranulocytosis/blood dyscrasias	•								⊛
Anticholinergic effects	•	•	•	•		•			⊛
Diabetes	•						•	•	⊛ ⑫
Dyslipidemia	•					•		•	⊛ ⑫
Extrapyramidal symptoms	•	•	•	•	•	•	•	•	⊛ ⑥
Hepatic effects	•			•					⊛
Neuroleptic malignant syndrome	•								⊛
Obesity/weight gain	•		•	•	•	•	•	•	⊛ ③
Ocular effects	•						•	•	⊛ ⑥
Prolactin effects	•			•		•	•	•	⊛ ⑥
QT prolongation/arrhythmias	•		•		•		•		⊛
Sedation/sleep disturbances	•	•	•	•	•		•		⊛
Seizures	•								⊛
Sexual dysfunction	•				•	•	•		⊛ ⑥
Sialorrhea	•								⊛
Skin/hypersensitivity reactions	•			•			•		⊛
Tardive dyskinesia	•					•	•	•	⊛ ⑥
Urinary incontinence	•			•					⊛
Venous thromboembolism	•								⊛
Vital signs	•	•	•	•	•	•	•	•	⊛ ⑥

• Monitor for adverse effect. ⊛ As clinically indicated. ③ Every 3 months. ⑥ Every 6 months. ⑫ Annually.

Notes: _____

_____

_____

Thiothixene

Monitoring schedule recommended for **THIOTHIXENE**

For specific monitoring recommendations related to each adverse effect, refer to the monitoring subheading of each chapter in Section 1.

	Baseline	Weeks 1	Weeks 2	Months 1	Months 2	Months 3	Months 6	Months 12	Long-term monitoring
Adverse effect									
Agranulocytosis/blood dyscrasias	•								(★)
Anticholinergic effects	•	Δ	•	Δ	Δ				(★)
Diabetes	•						•	•	(★) (12)
Dyslipidemia	•							•	(★) (12)
Extrapyramidal symptoms	•	•	•	•	•	•	•	•	(★) (6)
Hepatic effects	•			•					(★)
Neuroleptic malignant syndrome	•								(★)
Obesity/weight gain	•			•		•			(★) (6)
Ocular effects	•								(★)
Prolactin effects	•			•		•		•	(★) (6)
QT prolongation/arrhythmias	•		•		•		•		(★)
Sedation/sleep disturbances	•		•	•	•		•		(★)
Seizures	•								(★)
Sexual dysfunction	•					•		•	(★) (6)
Sialorrhea	•								(★)
Skin/hypersensitivity reactions	•			•			•		(★)
Tardive dyskinesia	•					•	•	•	(★) (6)
Urinary incontinence	•			•					(★)
Venous thromboembolism	•								(★)
Vital signs	•	•		•		•	•	•	(★) (6)

• Monitor for adverse effect. (★) As clinically indicated. (6) Every 6 months. (12) Annually. Δ Additional monitoring is recommended when an anticholinergic agent is co-prescribed with the antipsychotic.

Notes: _____

_____

_____

Trifluoperazine

Monitoring schedule recommended for **TRIFLUOPERAZINE**

For specific monitoring recommendations related to each adverse effect, refer to the monitoring subheading of each chapter in Section 1.

	Baseline	Weeks 1	Weeks 2	Months 1	Months 2	Months 3	Months 6	Months 12	Long-term monitoring
Adverse effect									
Agranulocytosis/blood dyscrasias	•								★
Anticholinergic effects	•	Δ	•	Δ	Δ				★
Diabetes	•						•	•	★ ⑫
Dyslipidemia	•					•		•	★ ⑫
Extrapyramidal symptoms	•	•	•	•	•	•	•	•	★ ⑥
Hepatic effects	•			•					★
Neuroleptic malignant syndrome	•								★
Obesity/weight gain	•				•		•		★ ⑥
Ocular effects	•						•	•	★ ⑥
Prolactin effects	•			•			•	•	★ ⑥
QT prolongation/arrhythmias	•		•		•				★
Sedation/sleep disturbances	•		•	•	•		•		★
Seizures	•								★
Sexual dysfunction	•					•	•	•	★ ⑥
Sialorrhea	•								★
Skin/hypersensitivity reactions	•				•		•		★
Tardive dyskinesia	•					•	•	•	★ ⑥
Urinary incontinence	•			•					★
Venous thromboembolism	•								★
Vital signs	•	•		•		•	•	•	★ ⑥

• Monitor for adverse effect. ★ As clinically indicated. ⑥ Every 6 months. ⑫ Annually. Δ Additional monitoring is recommended when an anticholinergic agent is co-prescribed with the antipsychotic.

Notes: _____

_____

_____

Ziprasidone

Monitoring schedule recommended for **ZIPRASIDONE**

For specific monitoring recommendations related to each adverse effect, refer to the monitoring subheading of each chapter in Section 1.

	Baseline	Weeks 1	Weeks 2	Months 1	Months 2	Months 3	Months 6	Months 12	Long-term monitoring
Adverse effect									
Agranulocytosis/blood dyscrasias	•								⊛
Anticholinergic effects	•								⊛
Diabetes	•						•	•	⊛ ⑫
Dyslipidemia	•					•		•	⊛ ⑫
Extrapyramidal symptoms	•		•	•		•		•	⊛ ⑥
Hepatic effects	•			•					⊛
Neuroleptic malignant syndrome	•								⊛
Obesity/weight gain	•			•		•	•	•	⊛ ⑥
Ocular effects	•								⊛
Prolactin effects	•								⊛
QT prolongation/arrhythmias	•		•		•		•		⊛
Sedation/sleep disturbances	•	•	•	•	•		•		⊛
Seizures	•								⊛
Sexual dysfunction	•					•	•	•	⊛ ⑥
Sialorrhea	•								⊛
Skin/hypersensitivity reactions	•			•			•		⊛
Tardive dyskinesia	•						•	•	⊛ ⑫
Urinary incontinence	•			•					⊛
Venous thromboembolism	•								⊛
Vital signs	•	•		•		•	•	•	⊛ ⑥

• Monitor for adverse effect. ⊛ As clinically indicated. ⑥ Every 6 months. ⑫ Annually.

Notes: _____

_____

_____

Zuclopenthixol

Monitoring schedule recommended for **ZUCLOPENTHIXOL**

For specific monitoring recommendations related to each adverse effect, refer to the monitoring subheading of each chapter in Section 1.

	Baseline	Weeks		Months					Long-term monitoring
		1	2	1	2	3	6	12	
Adverse effect									
Agranulocytosis/blood dyscrasias	•								★
Anticholinergic effects	•	Δ	•	Δ	Δ				★
Diabetes	•						•	•	★ ⑫
Dyslipidemia	•							•	★ ⑫
Extrapyramidal symptoms	•	•	•	•	•	•	•	•	★ ⑥
Hepatic effects	•			•					★
Neuroleptic malignant syndrome	•								★
Obesity/weight gain	•			•		•			★ ⑥
Ocular effects	•								★
Prolactin effects	•				•		•	•	★ ⑥
QT prolongation/arrhythmias	•		•		•		•		★
Sedation/sleep disturbances	•		•	•	•		•		★
Seizures	•								★
Sexual dysfunction	•					•	•	•	★ ⑥
Sialorrhea	•								★
Skin/hypersensitivity reactions	•			•			•		★
Tardive dyskinesia	•					•	•	•	★ ⑥
Urinary incontinence	•			•					★
Venous thromboembolism	•								★
Vital signs	•	•		•		•	•	•	★ ⑥

• Monitor for adverse effect. ★ As clinically indicated. ⑥ Every 6 months. ⑫ Annually. Δ Additional monitoring is recommended when an anticholinergic agent is co-prescribed with the antipsychotic.

Notes: _____

_____

_____

SECTION 3

General monitoring form for patients taking antipsychotics

Overview of the General Antipsychotic Monitoring Form

When screening and monitoring for side effects in patients taking antipsychotics long term, clinicians can benefit from thoughtfully designed and comprehensive monitoring forms that are easy to apply in daily practice. In this section, we have attempted to provide such a form along with a brief guide to its use.

With the General Antipsychotic Monitoring Form, we have attempted to distill the screening and monitoring recommendations from Sections 1 and 2 by creating a versatile monitoring tool. The form facilitates the systematic screening and monitoring of most antipsychotic side effects described in the book. It can be adapted by the user to meet specific monitoring needs, which will vary depending on patient characteristics and current antipsychotic treatment. The form provides general recommendations of when and what to monitor as well as the opportunity to document relevant findings succinctly. In this section, we provide a guide on its use. To address the concern that the monitoring recommendations may be too demanding, we encourage you try it out for three to five patients. We hope your ultimate decision about the value of the form will come from experiencing it.

If you would like to create copies of this form and/or would like to adapt it to your needs, it can be downloaded at **http://www.cambridge.org/9780521132084.**

Documentation of side effect screening and monitoring will be facilitated by routinely using the form in clinical practice. It is hoped that this will in turn lead to safer and more effective use of antipsychotics and will improve the overall care of patients taking antipsychotics long term.

As we mentioned in the Introduction (Chapter 1.1), patients with diagnoses of schizophrenia and bipolar disorder are at markedly increased risk of cardiovascular disease and cardiovascular death. Despite this, they are screened and monitored less often for risk factors and receive appropriate interventions less often than the general population. We also describe in the Introduction a general decline in the attention to movement disorders and the skills needed for assessing them. The General Antipsychotic Monitoring Form emphasizes screening and monitoring for these problems along with several other common or potentially serious adverse effects.

Frequently asked questions

The following six questions and answers are provided to help clarify when and how to use this form. Specific details describing the form's contents as well as how to use the form follow in Chapter 3.3.

1. Who should be monitored using this form?

Anyone receiving regular doses of an antipsychotic medication over weeks, months, or years.

2. When should this form be used?

This form should be used when a patient begins or is continuing on long-term antipsychotic treatment.

3. How should this form be used?

This will vary from one practice setting to the next. Some clinicians may use a replica of the form without any changes, while others may prefer to create their own form using ours as a starting point.

Ideally the form should be paired with and adapted to the monitoring schedule provided in Section 2 for the specific antipsychotic prescribed.

A form can be included in a patient's chart and referred to at each visit to ensure monitoring for side effects is a regular, structured part of patient care.

Responsibility for completing the form needs to be determined in advance for patients who have multiple health providers involved in their mental healthcare.

4. When should a new form be started?

Anytime a patient is started on a new antipsychotic medication. Also, begin a new form when the previous form has been completed.

5. How can I use the form for a patient who has been on an antipsychotic for quite some time?

Pages 180–181 are for patients who have been taking the same antipsychotic for <1 year.

Start with pages 182–184 if the patient has been on the antipsychotic for ≥1 year. At this point, screening and monitoring for antipsychotic side effects is usually scheduled every 3–6 months, as long as there are no ongoing issues that merit closer attention.

6. Should more than one form be used for patients on more than one antipsychotic?

No. Only one form per patient is necessary. Adapt the form as needed to ensure that appropriate monitoring occurs.

Pair the general monitoring form with the specific monitoring schedules of the antipsychotics prescribed (see Section 2).

Guide for using the General Antipsychotic Monitoring Form

Structure

The form has two pages, one for the first 12 months of antipsychotic treatment and the other for use after 12 months.

The upper sections of the form allow recording of specific patient and treatment information and development of a patient-specific schedule (which can be done "as you go"). Items to be monitored fall under the headings "Physical – general," "Assessment – special," and "Labs & other tests."

There are two types of cells in the form: filled cells and empty cells. The **filled cells**, which vary in their content (e.g. lines on which to record findings, indicators of normal [N] and abnormal [Abn]), indicate when in the schedule we encourage monitoring of the

specific item listed. The completely **empty cells** can be considered as optional dates for monitoring and documenting findings. Thus, these cells need not remain empty if the clinician feels that a test or assessment is warranted. The findings can be recorded in these cells. The final decision regarding what to monitor and when should be based on the specific antipsychotic prescribed (see suggested monitoring schedule in Section 2) and the patient's monitoring needs.

Content

The following examples of the form have been selected to provide guidance regarding how to use the monitoring tool most efficiently.

General Antipsychotic Monitoring Form: AP Year 1

Note: Inquire about other potential adverse effects as clinically indicated:	
• Cardiac disease indicators and risk factors • Ocular changes/vision problems • QT prolongation/arrhythmia indicator and risk factors • Seizures • Sialorrhea • Skin effects • Urinary incontinence • Venous thromboembolism indicators	A list of less common or unique but potentially serious and frequently unpredictable adverse effects require clinician awareness, monitoring, and investigation but are not included in the regular monitoring schedule of the form. Clinicians are to monitor for these as described in the respective chapters in Section 1.

SCHEDULE FOR YEAR 1*	Baseline	1 w	
Date planned*	___	___	**Date planned**: record on the lines provided the dates when the tests and assessments **should** be completed.
Date completed	___	___	**Date completed**: record the date when the tests and assessments **were** completed.

PHYSICAL - GENERAL	Baseline
Physical exam	N Abn
	Note:
Weight	———
BMI	———
Waist circumference	———
Blood pressure	L:———
	S:———
Heart rate	———
Temperature	

By circling N or Abn, record if the physical exam was normal or revealed any abnormalities. Beside Note: write the date of the medical chart entry in which the details of the exam were recorded.

For calculations and interpretations of BMI and waist circumference see Chapter 1.9.

Blood pressure: record lying (L) and standing (S) pressures.

Filled cells: are cells that use a line or text to suggest what tests or assessments should be completed and when.
Empty cells: are cells that are available for documenting results but whether or not to use this cell is at the clinician's discretion.

ASSESSMENT - SPECIAL	Baseline
Anticholinergic effects	N Abn
	Note:
EPS & TD	Ak __ Pk __
	Dk __ Dt __
Sedation/sleep inquiry	N Abn
	Note:
Prolactin inquiry	N Abn
	Note:
Sexual function inquiry	N Abn
	Note:
Diabetes symptom screen	N Abn
	Note:

Document the presence of akathisia (Ak), parkinsonism (Pk), dyskinesia (Dk), and dystonia (Dt). Use checkmarks, Y/N, or clinical global impression scores (see items V to VIII of the ESRS in Chapter 1.6).

For clinical inquiry and screening suggestions, refer to Chapters 1.4, 1.11, 1.13, and 1.15.

Circle N or Abn to indicate normal or abnormal findings. Use the Note to indicate the date the findings were documented in the chart for easy referral.

LABS & OTHER TESTS	Basline
Fasting plasma glucose	‾‾‾
A1C (if diabetes present)	
Hepatic effect (AST, ALT, ALP, GGT)	N Abn Lab:
Lipids	T-chol: ‾‾ LDL: ‾‾ HDL: ‾‾ T/H ratio TG: ‾‾
CBC[b]	N Abn Lab:
Prolactin	‾‾‾
ECG	N Abn Note:
Other	
Other	

On the line provided, document the test result. Add results into cells when additional relevant lab values known.

Record lipid profile. T-chol:HDL ratio is abbreviated T/H ratio and TG is triglycerides.

Record baseline FPG, hepatic test results, lipid profile, CBC, and if appropriate prolactin and ECG results. If abnormal (Abn), record the lab value and add follow-up findings in later empty cells.

If an ECG is completed, record it as normal (N) or abnormal (Abn) and Note the date of the recording, for easy retrieval.

Enter any other important monitoring relevant for a particular patient (e.g. EEG monitoring for a patient at high risk of seizures).

General Antipsychotic Monitoring Form: Ap Year ≥2

PHYSICAL - GENERAL	3 Month Intervals	
Physical exam	★ ⑫	
Weight	★ ③	‾‾
BMI	★ ③	‾‾
Waist circumference	★ ⑥	‾‾
Blood pressure	★ ⑫	
Heart rate	★ ⑫	
Temperature	★	

Use this page of the form for monitoring patients taking an antipsychotic for over a year.

The same symbols used in the book are applied here, indicating that monitoring is recommended every 3, 6, or 12 months, or as clinically indicated.

General Antipsychotic Monitoring Form: AP Year 1

Name:

DOB: Height:

Diagnosis:

Current antipsychotic(s):

Date started:

Past antipsychotics:

Comments:

Note: Inquire about other potential adverse effects as clinically indicated:

- Cardiac disease indicators and risk factors
- Ocular changes/vision problems
- QT prolongation/arrhythmia indicators and risk factors
- Seizures
- Sialorrhea
- Skin effects
- Urinary incontinence
- Venous thromboembolism indicators

SCHEDULE FOR YEAR 1[a]	Baseline	1 week	2 weeks	1 month	2 months	3 months	6 months	12 months
Date planned[a]								
Date completed								

PHYSICAL – GENERAL	Baseline	1 week	2 weeks	1 month	2 months	3 months	6 months	12 months
Physical exam	N Abn Note:							N Abn Note:
Weight								
BMI								
Waist circumference								
Blood pressure	L: S:	L: S:		L: S:		L: S:	L: S:	
Heart rate								
Temperature								

ASSESSMENT – SPECIAL	Baseline	1 week	2 weeks	1 month	2 months	3 months	6 months	12 months
Anticholinergic effects	N Abn Note:		N Abn Note:	N Abn Note:	N Abn Note:		N Abn Note:	N Abn Note:
EPS and TD	Ak___ Pk___ Dk___ Dt___		Ak___ Pk___ Dk___ Dt___	Ak___ Pk___ Dk___ Dt___	Ak___ Pk___ Dk___ Dt___	Ak___ Pk___ Dk___ Dt___	Ak___ Pk___ Dk___ Dt___	Ak___ Pk___ Dk___ Dt___

LABS & OTHER TESTS [inquiries]	Baseline	1 week	2 weeks	1 month	2 months	3 months	6 months	12 months
Sedation/sleep inquiry	N Abn / Note:		N Abn / Note:		N Abn / Note:		N Abn / Note:	N Abn / Note:
Prolactin inquiry	N Abn / Note:			N Abn / Note:		N Abn / Note:	N Abn / Note:	N Abn / Note:
Sexual function inquiry	N Abn / Note:					N Abn / Note:	N Abn / Note:	N Abn / Note:
Diabetes symptom screen	N Abn / Note:						N Abn / Note:	N Abn / Note:
LABS & OTHER TESTS	**Baseline**	**1 week**	**2 weeks**	**1 month**	**2 months**	**3 months**	**6 months**	**12 months**
Fasting plasma glucose	____						____	
A1C (if diabetes present)								
Hepatic effects (AST, ALT, ALP, GGT)	N Abn / Lab:			N Abn / Lab:				
Lipids	T-chol: ____ / LDL: ____ / HDL: ____ / T/H ratio: ____ / TG: ____					T-chol: ____ / LDL: ____ / HDL: ____ / T/H ratio: ____ / TG: ____		T-chol: ____ / LDL: ____ / HDL: ____ / T/H ratio: ____ / TG: ____
CBC[b]	N Abn / Lab:							
Prolactin								
ECG	N Abn / Note:							
Other								
Other								

A1C = glycated hemoglobin; Abn = abnormal; Ak = akathisia; ALP = alkaline phosphatase; ALT = alanine transaminase; AP = antipsychotic; AST = aspartate transaminase; CBC = complete blood count; Dk = dyskinesia; Dt = dystonia; ECG = electrocardiogram; EPS = extrapyramidal symptoms; GGT = gamma glutamyltransferase; HDL = high-density lipoprotein; L = lying; LDL = low-density lipoprotein; N = normal; Pk = parkinsonism; S = standing; TD = tardive dyskinesia; T-chol = total cholesterol; TG = triglycerides; T/H ratio = ratio of total cholesterol:HDL cholesterol values.

[a] Adapt the monitoring schedule and related documentation based on the antipsychotic prescribed (see Section 2) and patient-specific issues.
[b] Clozapine requires special monitoring.

Source: Gardner DM and Teehan MD. *Antipsychotics and their Side Effects*. Cambridge University Press, 2011. © DM Gardner and MD Teehan 2011. Available at: http://www.cambridge.org/9780521132084.

General Antipsychotic Monitoring Form: AP Year ≥2

Name: _____

DOB: _____ Height: _____

Diagnosis: _____

Current antipsychotic(s): _____

Date started: _____

Past antipsychotics: _____

Comments: _____

Note: Inquire about other potential adverse effects as clinically indicated:
- Cardiac disease indicators and risk factors
- Ocular changes/vision problems
- QT prolongation/arrhythmia indicators and risk factors
- Seizures
- Sialorrhea
- Skin effects
- Urinary incontinence
- Venous thromboembolism indicators

SCHEDULE FOR YEAR ≥2[a]	3-Month intervals							
Date planned[a]								
Date completed								

PHYSICAL – GENERAL	3-Month intervals							
Physical exam (★) (12)			N Abn Note:				N Abn Note:	
Weight (★) (3)								
BMI (★) (3)								
Waist circumference (★) (6)								
Blood pressure (★) (6)			L: ____ S: ____				L: ____ S: ____	
Heart rate (★) (6)								
Temperature (★)								

ASSESSMENT – SPECIAL	3-Month intervals							
Anticholinergic effects (★)								

EPS & TD ⋆ ⑥	Ak___ Pk___ Dk___ Dt___	Ak___ Pk___ Dk___ Dt___	Ak___ Pk___ Dk___ Dt___	Ak___ Pk___ Dk___ Dt___
Sedation/sleep inquiry ⋆				
Prolactin inquiry ⋆ ⑫	N Abn Note:		N Abn Note:	N Abn Note:
Sexual function inquiry ⋆ ⑥	N Abn Note:	N Abn Note:	N Abn Note:	N Abn Note:
Diabetes symptom screen ⋆ ⑫	N Abn Note:		N Abn Note:	N Abn Note:

LABS & OTHER TESTS — 3-Month intervals

Fasting plasma glucose ⋆ ⑫	___		___	___
A1C (if diabetes present) ⋆				
Hepatic effects (AST, ALT, ALP, GGT) ⋆				
Lipids ⋆ ⑫	T-chol: ___ LDL: ___ HDL: ___ T/H ratio: ___ TG: ___		T-chol: ___ LDL: ___ HDL: ___ T/H ratio: ___ TG: ___	T-chol: ___ LDL: ___ HDL: ___ T/H ratio: ___ TG: ___
CBC[b] ⋆				
Prolactin ⋆				
ECG ⋆				
Other				
Other				

(★) As clinically indicated. (3) Every 3 months. (6) Every 6 months. (12) Annually.

A1C = glycated hemoglobin; Abn = abnormal; Ak = akathisia; ALP = alkaline phosphatase; ALT = alanine transaminase; AP = antipsychotic; AST = aspartate transaminase; CBC = complete blood count; Dk = dyskinesia; Dt = dystonia; ECG = electrocardiogram; EPS = extrapyramidal symptoms; GGT = gamma glutamyltransferase; HDL = high-density lipoprotein; L = lying; LDL = low-density lipoprotein; N = normal; Pk = parkinsonism; S = standing; TD = tardive dyskinesia; T-chol = total cholesterol; TG = triglycerides; T/H ratio = ratio of total cholesterol:HDL cholesterol values.

[a] Adapt the monitoring schedule and related documentation based on the antipsychotic prescribed (see source Section 2) and patient-specific issues.

[b] Clozapine requires special monitoring.

Source: Gardner DM and Teehan MD. *Antipsychotics and their Side Effects.* Cambridge University Press, 2011. © DM Gardner and MD Teehan 2011. Available at: http://www.cambridge.org/9780521132084.

Index